Keven,

I am blessed with the opportunity to work with you to minister to our residents. Thank you for your dedication to our shared goals. Jamie Lange

Enhancing
Staff Retention
in Person-Centered
Care Environments
for Older Adults

Enhancing Staff Retention in Person-Centered Care Environments for Older Adults

How to Create and Implement a Comprehensive Orientation Program

by
Janine M. Lange, M.S.N., R.N.-B.C.

Foreword by
Vickie G. Rodgers, M.S.N., R.N.-B.C.

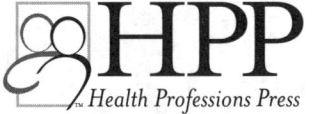
HPP
Health Professions Press

Baltimore • London • Sydney

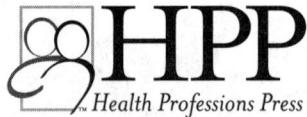

Health Professions Press, Inc.
Post Office Box 10624
Baltimore, Maryland 21285-0624

www.healthpropress.com

Interior and cover designs by Mindy Dunn.
Typeset by Mindy Dunn.
Manufactured in the United States of America by Maple Press, York, Pennsylvania.

Library of Congress Cataloging-in-Publication Data

Lange, Janine M., author.
  Enhancing staff retention in person-centered care environments for older adults : how to create and implement a comprehensive orientation program / by Janine M. Lange ; foreword by Vickie G. Rodgers.
     p. ; cm.
  Includes index.
  ISBN 978-1-938870-41-5 (pbk.)
  I. Title.
  [DNLM: 1. In-service Training—methods. 2. Nursing Staff—education. 3. Homes for the Aged—organization & administration. 4. Nursing Homes—organization & administration. 5. Patient-Centered Care—organization & administration. WX 159]
  RT120.L64
  362.16071'55—dc23
                              2015030601

British Library Cataloguing-in-Publication data are available from the British Library.
E-book Edition: ISBN 978-1-938870-51-4

*I dedicate this book first and foremost to my husband Daniel,
whose love, support, and encouragement helped me realize
my potential and attain my dreams. Second, to the finest
hospice nurse I know who taught me everything about putting
the care of others above all else, my mother.*

*I also dedicate this book to my dad, who always believed in me,
encouraged me, and told me to "be successful in anything
you endeavor to do." And to my dearest friend Tracy,
who may have lost the battle, but never lost hope.*

*And finally, to my colleagues, who have chosen to follow in
the footsteps of nursing pioneers to bring hope and healing to others.*

Contents

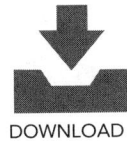

DOWNLOAD

Downloadable Resources

The following sample agendas, checklists, and forms are available for download at www.healthpropress.com/lange-downloads (use password [case sensitive]: GE9K2X3).

Nursing Department Orientation Program Agenda

Nursing Orientation Program Checklist

Privacy and Protected Information Compliance Form

Mentor Agreement

Mentor Application Form

Mentor Training Agenda

Supervisor Recommendation Form for Mentor Program

Tiered Compensation Plan for Mentors

Skills Demonstration Checklist

Medication Administration Test

Skills Demonstration Checklist (CNA/CMT)

Skills Demonstration Checklist (RN/LPN)

Resident Transfer Training Checklist

Gait Belt Compliance Form

"Take Me Out to the Ballgame" Annual Skills Fair Day

The Story of Me

Nursing Orientation Evaluation Form

30- to 60-Day Mentorship Evaluation Form

About the Author

Janine Lange, M.S.N., R.N.-B.C., began her nursing career in Billings, Montana, as a respite care volunteer for seniors in her community. She quickly developed a passion for caring for others, especially those with life-threatening illnesses, and became a registered nurse. After acquiring experience in the hospital setting, Lange devoted her nursing career to being a hospice nurse, having witnessed the loving care her father received from the nurses at a Veterans Health Administration hospital, where he succumbed to the ravages of lung cancer.

Following additional training in nursing management and administration, including earning certification as a Staff Development Specialist in Long-Term Care, Lange became Director of Clinical Education for one of the top 10, not-for-profit continuing care retirement communities in the United States. She focuses on improving the training process for new nursing staff and providing continuing education to help staff hone their skills.

An advocate for the rights of residents and the education of those who care for them, Lange is a leader in culture change and supporting the values and practices of person-centered care. As a speaker for national conventions and nursing organizations, she stresses the importance of comprehensive orientation training to improve staff retention and performance. She is also actively involved in the Pioneer Network, an organization that advocates for culture change across all models of elder care and elder services.

Foreword

Long-term care has always been a great passion for both Janine and me. Together we have collaborated on many educational projects to enhance care, improve staffing consistency, and support continuing education for staff in long-term care. Janine's dedication to promoting resident and staff well-being is matched equally by her brilliance in designing highly effective training programs for care teams. Both talents are reflected in this excellent resource that will dramatically enhance the implementation of person-centered care practices in any long-term care setting.

Many long-term care communities are adopting person-centered care approaches to improve the overall quality of life for their residents as well as the job satisfaction of their employees. Maintaining consistent staffing is crucial in providing person-centered care, and a good orientation program that includes a strong mentoring component is essential to this goal.

In my previous role as a long-term care clinical nurse educator, I had implemented this orientation program with our newly hired nursing staff. The program proved very effective in creating an environment where new staff feel welcomed and valued. Additionally, the extended training period allows new nursing staff time to develop their skills and to better understand the overall person-centered care environment. The adoption of this comprehensive orientation program resulted in increased staff satisfaction and, as a result, increased staff retention rates.

For many years, long-term care has endured a high turnover rate in nursing staff, with minimal or even dismal orientations and no consistent mentoring of new employees. This is in contrast to the acute care environment, where nursing staff are given 6–12 weeks of orientation as well as the luxury of a consistently assigned mentor.

In *Enhancing Staff Retention in Person-Centered Care Environments for Older Adults*, Janine Lange provides a wealth of information to nurse educators, directors of nursing, administrators, and human resources directors in long-term care to help them develop effective and sustainable orientation training and mentoring programs that welcome new team members to the community and that set them up for success in delivering person-centered care to residents. I believe you will find this book to be a valuable resource in your care of older adults.

Vickie G. Rodgers, M.S.N., R.N.-B.C.
Associate Professor of Nursing
Lewis and Clark Community College
Godfrey, Illinois

Preface

Having the reputation as a preferred employer attracts top-quality employees who are enthusiastic and dedicated and who possess an exceptional work ethic. Typically, an organization stands above the rest not only because of the excellent care they provide, but also as a result of staff satisfaction and retention. This book is a guide for creating a comprehensive orientation program to help communities of all sizes train and retain staff and, thereby, become an employer of choice.

A well-developed, person-centered orientation program is the first step to integrating new team members into the culture of a community and setting them on the path to success. Drawing on my experiences as a Clinical Nurse Educator and Director of Nursing, I have written this book to help communities avoid the challenges of a high rate of staff turnover, the consequences of deficient annual state surveys, and the negative outcomes associated with providing substandard care to residents.

Fundamentally, the needs of new staff are the same: They require clear and concise information about the organization, its culture and mission, and the expectations of supervisors. They also require a thorough education in all aspects of their job. This book covers these key topics and provides the tools necessary to create a comprehensive orientation program specific to your organization, including sample agendas, checklists, and forms that can be modified and personalized. The book also discusses the benefits of providing good mentoring to new team members and shows you how to begin your own mentor training program.

Residents and families have many choices in long-term care. Knowing that your community is vigilant about maintaining a well-educated, culturally sensitive team of caregivers will influence their selection process. How an organization welcomes and trains new employees speaks volumes about their commitment to the success of their staff. *Enhancing Staff Retention in Person-Centered Care Environments for Older Adults* will help you prepare your team members to provide the caliber of care consumers expect for their loved ones.

My vision is for all healthcare communities to work hand-in-hand with their team members to provide outstanding, person-centered care to their residents. I have been inspired by my fellow nurses, educators, nurse aides, and nurse managers in developing the contents of this book. We share a common bond in our dedication to caring for others, and our success lies in the knowledge that we make a difference in their lives each and every day. I wish the same joy and satisfaction for you and your staff.

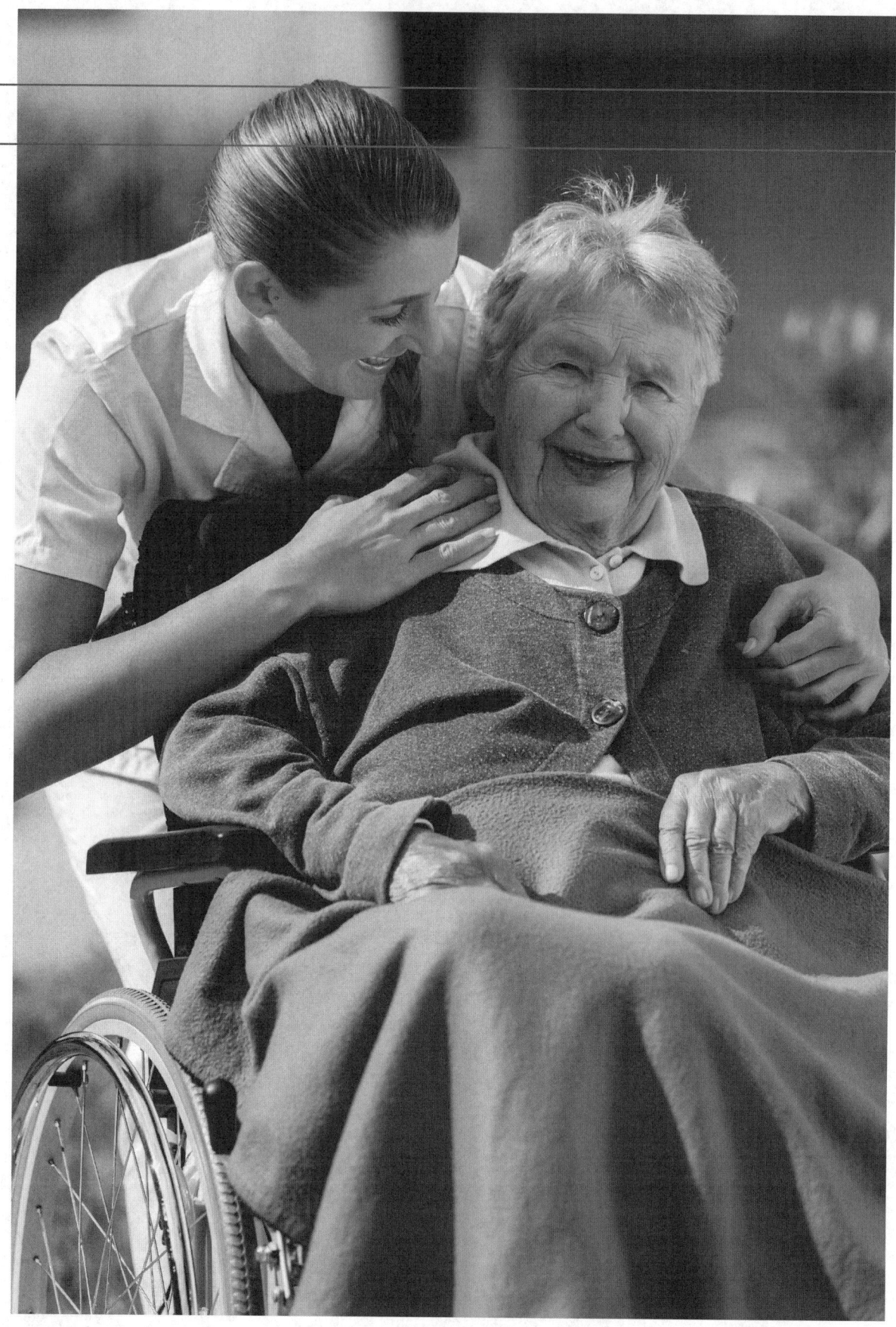

Introduction

One of the most challenging aspects of providing person-centered care is assembling a dedicated, competent, and well-trained team of caregivers. Continuity of care is compromised when there is a high rate of employee turnover; it is detrimental to the well-being of the residents and is a financial burden to the employer. Constant hiring and rehiring degrades the integrity of the staff and diminishes the reputation of a long-term care community.

The orientation process for our caregivers is one of the most important investments of time and resources we can make and is absolutely essential to ensure your residents will receive the care they deserve. After the initial processes of interviewing and hiring are completed, it is imperative to prepare your new team members to become an integral part of your community. Providing an in-depth, comprehensive orientation program will equip new team members with the tools needed to be successful.

As a former Director of Nursing, I understand firsthand the critical consequences of allowing staff who are unprepared, insecure, and not properly trained to provide care to residents. My role as Director of Clinical Education has afforded me the opportunity to address these dangerous situations and help prepare our nursing staff to develop and enhance their skills as they strive each and every day to have a profound impact on our residents.

This book will guide you through the process of creating a person-centered orientation program that will suit your specific needs and set you on the path to forming long-lasting relationships with your staff and the residents they serve. Your community will reap the benefits of placing the safety and well-being of your residents in the capable hands and caring hearts of their caregivers.

ABOUT THE *NEIGHBORHOOD*

Throughout the book, you will notice that I often use the terms *Neighborhood* or *Household*. The community in which I work embraces culture change and strives to deliver person-centered care. To create a home-like atmosphere for our residents, we prefer the terms *Neighborhood* or *Household* as opposed to *unit* or *hall*. All of our Neighborhoods are named after distinctive St. Louis landmarks, such as Laclede's Landing, Ball Park Village, Kiener Plaza, and so forth. There are pictures of each landmark throughout the Neighborhoods to make it easier for residents to distinguish one area from another and also to help them recognize where they live.

The difference between a Neighborhood and Household is that a Household has fewer residents, usually 10 to 15, whereas a Neighborhood is larger with about 18 to 22 residents. Each area is self-sufficient with its own kitchen, living room, dining room, nurses' desk, laundry room, and so forth. All of the meals are prepared on each Neighborhood to help stimulate appetites and enhance the dining experience. Additionally, in keeping with the true essence of culture change and a person-centered care approach, each Neighborhood or Household has a team of designated, consistent staff to help build relationships between the residents and their caregivers.

ABOUT THE BOOK

Chapter 1 discusses the first steps in developing an orientation program—identifying the needs of your community and then choosing the topics to present in support of addressing those needs. The chapter also identifies 12 key components that should form the basis of the program and that will increase the likelihood of success in training new staff members. Chapter 2 reviews the process of creating an agenda for the orientation program, including prioritizing the topics to be presented, identifying time allotments for agenda items and taking breaks, and listing the names and titles of those who will present specific topics. Chapter 3 discusses the importance of building and maintaining a successful mentor program in support of the orientation process. A solid mentoring program will provide a consistent method of teaching that extends beyond the first few days and weeks in the Neighborhood and will also identify and promote the future leaders in your organization.

Chapter 4 emphasizes the need to educate orientees to the various staff titles and responsibilities in the Neighborhood that reflect your community's person-centered care practice, as well as the importance of building relationships with residents and co-workers. For those new hires who are unfamiliar with a person-centered care approach, defining the culture of your community is essential during training. Chapter 5 outlines how to conduct the orientation program, including preparing the classroom, making introductions, reviewing the agenda, and taking a walking tour of the Neighborhood with the new team members. Chapter 6 discusses the importance of skills testing in developing and enhancing the skills of new and existing nursing staff and the need for continuing education.

Chapter 7 offers tips for welcoming new staff during their first few weeks in the Neighborhood as they become familiar with existing staff and their surroundings and as the mentor–mentee relationship develops. Chapter 8 focuses further on the person-centered care approach by emphasizing the need for new staff to build relationships with residents, families, and existing staff as a way of building a trusting and caring environment. The chapter also offers techniques to enhance communication with residents, including the use of conversation starters. Chapter 9 addresses the importance of recognizing and welcoming the cultural diversity of new staff as well as providing additional help to those who speak English as a second language, to avoid potential issues in communicating with residents. Equally as important is the need for your community to acknowledge the traditions and customs that residents and staff observe, to strengthen relationships between staff and residents and among team members.

Chapter 10 discusses the need for nursing team members to maintain a connection and line of communication with new hires to make them feel welcomed and cared about during their first few weeks working in the Neighborhood alongside their mentor. The evaluation process for orientees is reviewed in Chapter 11, including how to create evaluation forms, when evaluations should be performed, and who should be involved. Chapter 12 examines five common barriers that detract from successfully forming long-lasting employer–employee relationships. Finally, Chapter 13 discusses the heart of the matter in developing a successful orientation program—first and foremost addressing the needs of residents.

The end of each chapter includes a summary review of the key topics covered as well as space at the bottom of the page to include your own notes. Several chapters also include sample forms and checklists that are discussed in the text. All of the forms and checklists are suitable for copying for ease of use and are also available for download by logging on to www.healthpropress.com/lange-downloads (use password [case sensitive]: GE9K2X3).

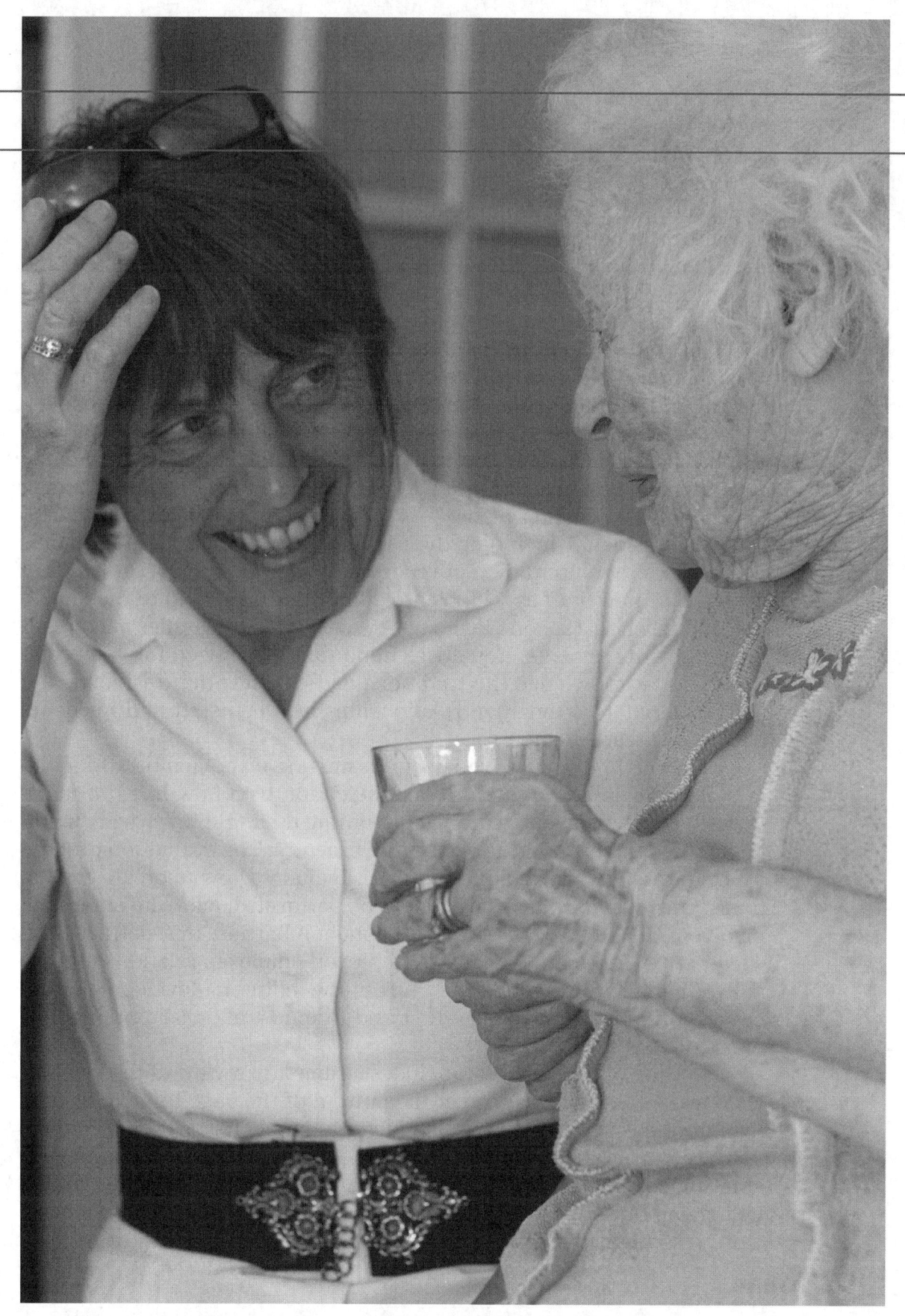

CHAPTER 1

Establish the Needs of Your Community

The success of any healthcare organization lies largely in the hands and hearts of the staff who have direct contact with residents and guests. Every employer strives to build and maintain a dedicated team who is caring, compassionate, and proficient in their skills and abilities. In a person-centered care environment, the emphasis is on building relationships and creating a sense of family with residents, their loved ones, and co-workers. A well-prepared orientation program introduces new team members to your culture and helps them become an integral part of your community.

To build a successful orientation program, you must begin by identifying the needs of your community. Person-centered care places a high priority on continuity and consistency in staffing to achieve optimum resident satisfaction. The community's goals should be to maintain a reliable team of employees, minimize the rate of employee turnover, and develop and enhance relationships between residents and staff. Objectively evaluate your present situation when developing a plan to train and retain staff by soliciting feedback from residents and staff through satisfaction surveys. This process can provide key information as to how your community may be struggling and which areas need improvement.

The Human Resources department can furnish statistics on the number of staff hired in a 12-month period and the longevity of current staff. If exit interviews are performed when an employee leaves your community, it is important to learn the reasons why he or she decided to leave. Ask specific questions about the factors leading to his or her decision and use this information to identify potential changes that may better promote employee retention.

Analyzing staffing patterns is important when evaluating quality and consistency. Determine how often PRN staff (i.e., staff called in as needed) or agency personnel are being used, since neither of these options lend themselves to good resident-to-staff relationships and should be used only as a last resort. By aligning your needs and goals, you can begin to build your orientation program in a manner that will increase the likelihood of success.

The contents of a comprehensive orientation program will vary depending on the requirements of each individual organization. The core of the program, however, should be comprised of the following 12 essential components:

1. Departmental education
2. Products and services
3. Culture change and person-centered care
4. Electronic medical records training
5. Alzheimer's and dementia training
6. Abuse and neglect and resident dignity
7. Accidents and injuries
8. Skills testing
9. Admission and discharge process
10. Infection control
11. Reducing return-to-hospital rates
12. Evaluations

DEPARTMENTAL EDUCATION

This section contains information specific to the Nursing department not covered in the general Human Resources orientation. Here you will discuss your dress code policy, which may be different in a person-centered care environment. Most person-centered care communities have moved away from scrubs or uniforms, preferring instead casual dress. This creates a more home-like atmosphere and is less likely to resemble an acute care setting. There are boundaries that must be specified to staff, such as whether employees are allowed to wear jeans, whether shirts must have collars, if only specific colored clothing is allowed, what is considered appropriate footwear (e.g., shoes that are closed-toed and heeled), and so forth. Include your policy on hair restraints. Since many communities prepare food in the Neighborhood, hairnets may be required. Discuss fingernail restrictions, including length, cleanliness, and artificial versus natural nails. Include your policy on tattoos and piercings as well.

The Nursing department generally works different shifts from other departments. Define the hours of work for each shift, including meal times and breaks. Review the differences between full-time, part-time, and PRN staff. Explain the procedure for call-ins, overtime, weekend options, paid time off, holidays, and pay periods. The scheduler can explain how each schedule is created, how often it repeats itself, and how to request changes. Depending on your community's protocol, all questions related to schedules should be directed to the scheduler. He or she should identify the preferred method of contact, such as in writing or via email or voice mail, and the expected response time. Also, the scheduler should state the amount of advance notice needed for time off requests, such as 2 weeks prior to the date(s) requested as time off.

Direct the orientees to the location of the time clock. Provide instruction on the procedure to follow if one forgets to clock in. This is also a good time to explain your on-time rules and attendance guidelines. Point out the staff parking area and whether parking tags are required to be displayed in the vehicle. Provide a map of the community showing all areas, including the business office, Human Resources department, cafeteria, laundry, housekeeping, and so forth.

PRODUCTS AND SERVICES

As part of this section, you will present the various products and services that your community provides. List and discuss the skin care products used in your community. Most skin care companies make available DVDs or videos to show how each product is used. Include instructions and tips for using each product. During the orientation program let the orientees try the lotions and cleansers to experience how they feel on the skin. Stress the importance of proper skin care for residents and the consequences of poor pericare and skin care.

Review in detail the incontinence products, including any toileting or trial programs used in your community. Wound care products and services and the policies and protocols that accompany them should also be thoroughly reviewed. Show pictures, slide presentations, or videos depicting different types of wounds and the appropriate products to use for treatments. Again, most companies provide training videos to demonstrate the proper use of their products.

Educate new team members about the different types of services your company employs, such as the pharmacy, labs, oxygen, and X-rays. Include the method of contact for ordering services and the required paperwork. Discuss adjunct services, such as physical therapy, hospice, home health, dialysis, podiatry, dental care, skin and wound care, or psychiatric care. Make sure the contact information is readily accessible and up to date.

CULTURE CHANGE AND PERSON-CENTERED CARE

In this section, describe where the community is on the path to culture change. Describe the structure of the Neighborhoods or Households. Define the roles each team member plays in the daily operations of the Neighborhood. You may choose to give a brief history of your organization and community showing advances and changes that have been made to enhance the living experiences of residents. If your community is in the beginning stages of culture change, describe your goals and plans toward transformation. As part of the orientation program, invite new team members to share their own personal experiences with person-centered care.

Discuss the ways in which your community honors person-centered care, such as:

- giving residents choices in bed, meal, and bath times as well as when medications are administered
- providing activities based on residents' requests and desires
- offering alternative choices to pharmaceutical interventions to address resident challenging behaviors
- building relationships between staff and the residents and family members they serve
- promoting and enhancing resident self-determination
- enforcing a consistent staffing policy

ELECTRONIC MEDICAL RECORDS TRAINING

New staff will come from a wide variety of experiences and expertise in charting. Most hospitals, sub-acute care settings, and long-term care communities use electronic medical records (EMR) for charting. Although the basic principles will be similar, there are many different electronic charting programs. It is important to recognize each orientee's level of comfort with EMR charting; therefore, ample time should be allowed when teaching your community's EMR program.

Emphasize from the beginning that the training class is only meant to be an introduction to the EMR system and additional training will take place in the Neighborhood. The EMR class should be taught by someone who is an expert, or super user, of the system. If resources allow, have a computer or laptop available for every one to two orientees so they can experience hands-on training. If your EMR system has a training environment, walk the orientees through the process of admitting a new resident and entering orders. Have a case study available for practice. Include instruction on entering items such as allergies, advance directives, personal and demographic information, immunizations, activities of daily living, therapy needs, dietary needs, and so forth. Prepare mock examples of a variety of orders and show how to enter them correctly.

While training on the EMR system, this is an opportune time to review your community's policy on passwords and electronic signatures. Stress the importance of keeping passwords private and that no one should ever be allowed to chart under someone else's name or password. Reiterate the legal aspect of charting in the resident's record and the consequences of poor or inaccurate information. For example, if a resident's chart were to be used in court for litigation, a nurse's documentation would serve as the only written account of what occurred during the resident's stay. Incomplete or missing documentation could be interpreted as not having been done. The following is an example of missing documentation:

a.	A resident's vital signs were recorded as "Blood Pressure 76/44."
b.	No follow-up treatment was documented after the vital signs were taken, such as rechecking the blood pressure, adjusting medications, and/or notifying the physician.
c.	The resident fell and suffered a hematoma to the head.
d.	The resident passed away as a result of his injuries.

In this situation, a nurse could be held liable for negligence because the documentation did not prove any subsequent action was taken after an abnormal vital sign was detected. Even if the nurse did follow through, there is no written proof.

ALZHEIMER'S AND DEMENTIA TRAINING

New team members from every level of care should receive training on Alzheimer's and dementia. Content should include recognizing different forms of communication, previously referred to as "behaviors," and how to deal with them. Verify your state regulations on the number of hours of dementia training required as it varies not only from state to state, but from assisted living to long-term care environments as well.

Role-playing is an excellent way to have staff experience some of the difficulties residents face on a daily basis. One exercise is to write a feeling or command on a piece of paper, such as "I am lonely" or "I need to use the restroom." Pair up orientees and give one person the slip of paper. Have him or her convey the message to his or her partner without speaking. Often, the person trying to understand the message becomes upset and frustrated trying to comprehend what is being asked of him or her. By putting themselves in the resident's place, this type of sensitivity training helps new staff understand the feelings residents experience each and every day. Another excellent exercise is to have the orientees spend time in a wheelchair with earplugs that mute their hearing and glasses that distort their vision. Let them try to navigate their way through the Neighborhood so they can fully grasp the difficulties and frustrations residents endure by not being mobile or able to hear or see well. Follow these exercises with suggestions for how to communicate with residents who have Alzheimer's or dementia, including the following:

- Position yourself close to the resident at his or her level.
- Never stand over the resident.
- Give the resident ample response time.
- Make eye contact with the resident.
- Do not offer the resident too many choices.
- Keep noise and commotion to a minimum.
- Use gestures in addition to verbal cues to help the resident understand.
- Speak clearly and slowly when addressing the resident.

ABUSE AND NEGLECT AND RESIDENT DIGNITY

Spell out your community's policies on abuse, neglect, and resident dignity, including definitions and reporting procedures. Reinforce the different types of abuse that can occur, such as verbal, physical, mental, sexual, and monetary abuse and involuntary seclusion. Videos are an excellent way to train new team members how to recognize abuse and how to provide care in a dignified manner because the portrayals are often accurate and leave a lasting impression on those who view them. Staff may not understand that separating a resident who is loud and disruptive from the dining room and confining the person to his or her room is a form of abuse. Neglect can be construed as walking past a resident who is asking for help without stopping to see what he or she needs. Neglect can also be the act of not using a gait belt with a resident who is unable to transfer independently. These are all examples of abuse and neglect that are often discounted and are never acceptable.

Cultural, age, and gender differences can play a role in issues with maintaining dignity during care. To an older gentleman, it is embarrassing and undignified to have personal care performed by a young, female nurse or aide. Staff should be sensitive to these feelings and provide care accordingly. Perhaps having a male aide or nurse tend to the resident will ease his discomfort and maintain his sense of dignity. Most caregivers have never experienced using a bedside commode in the presence of others or have never bathed in a large shower room with little or no privacy. Heightening caregivers' awareness of different aspects of dignity will help them provide care in a dignified manner.

ACCIDENTS AND INJURIES

Although communities strive to keep their residents free from falls or injuries of any type, it is inevitable that they will occur. In this section explain your community's policies on preventative measures for falls as well as the procedure to follow when a fall, accident, or injury occurs. To help guide new staff through the process, create a checklist with the items to be covered in the training, beginning first and foremost with providing care for the resident. Include appropriate interventions that may be implemented when a resident falls in order to prevent additional falls. Provide training on thorough and complete documentation of the incident and emphasize the potential legal ramifications in the event an accident or injury results in a court case. It is good practice to have a representative from the Risk Management or Legal department of your organization address this topic.

Accidents and injuries pertain not only to residents, but to staff and guests as well. Provide instruction on your company's process for handling such events. Include how and where to send injured persons who require medical attention, such as to a clinic or emergency room, as well as the paperwork that must be completed. Since workers' compensation may play a part in any employee-related injury that occurs while on the job, make sure new hires clearly understand the process. A representative from the Human Resources department would be a suitable speaker for this topic as part of the orientation program.

SKILLS TESTING

Every new team member, whether he or she has years of experience or is newly licensed, should be skills tested before stepping out into the Neighborhood to begin working with residents. Start by referring to your policy and procedure manual to ensure staff are performing services in accordance with your community's specific guidelines. Seasoned nurses, especially those coming from a different area of nursing, may not be aware of recommended long-term care practices. New graduates without any prior experience will benefit greatly from a skills testing class to help them gain confidence and enhance their capabilities.

Create tests for each discipline that are specific to the individual scope of practice. For certified nursing assistants (CNA), use the skills checklists from your state's CNA training manual. Check for current updates if the procedures have not been revised for several years. Certified medication technician (CMT) and nurse competency tests can be created with the assistance of your pharmacy since they will have the most up-to-date information on medication administration.

ADMISSION AND DISCHARGE PROCESS

One of the more stressful situations a new team member encounters is a new admission. The detailed paperwork, assessments, order entries, and care plans that must be completed and processes that must be performed correctly are extensive. Provide an admission checklist that itemizes each step in order of importance to be completed within the first 24 hours of a new resident's stay in your community. This will take the guesswork out of the process and ensure nothing gets overlooked. Review each item on the checklist in detail with new team members, including instructions for the following:

- where to document information in the electronic medical record
- how to create a care plan
- how to verify and enter an order
- where to send admission paperwork
- how to document skin and wound issues
- how to complete a do-not-resuscitate (DNR) order or full code documentation

The admission checklist will most likely be several pages long, but it is a necessary tool for both new as well as current staff. During the mentoring process (Chapter 3), it is best practice to have the new hire observe an admission or discharge.

The most important goal to stress to new team members about admissions is to always maintain a person-centered atmosphere and approach to the process. Encourage orientees to remind themselves to consider the feelings of the new resident and understand that this can be a stressful and difficult time for the person and his or her family members. Although there is an abundance of paperwork and assessments to perform, staff must be observant for signs that the resident is tiring, hungry, or may need to use the restroom. Provide rest intervals during the process. If the resident has endured a long trip from the hospital or home, have a small snack or drink available for him or her. If necessary, take a break and re-approach later when the person has had time to adjust to the changes. Staff should also be mindful of family members' feelings, especially if they are having difficulty accepting the fact that a parent or loved one is now living in a long-term care community.

The discharge process should be completed in the same manner for residents who are either going home or to a hospital. Once again, train new team members to use a checklist to ensure the process is accurate and complete.

When a death occurs at the community, explain the procedure to the orientees, including details on the following matters:

- who is qualified to pronounce the death
- necessary notifications (physician; family; hospice, if applicable; chaplain; medical examiner or coroner)
- organ donor notification process, if applicable
- calling the funeral home
- vital information to include in documentation
- medication returns and/or narcotics destruction
- notification of appropriate durable medical equipment company

INFECTION CONTROL

The infection control portion of the orientation program should include a detailed description of your community's policies and procedures, with special attention given to standard precautions and isolation. Explain how team members handle residents with C-Difficile, VRE, pneumonia, flu, and other communicable diseases. Describe the proper use and location of personal protective equipment (PPE). Have each new team member demonstrate proper technique for donning and removing PPE. You may choose to use a video or PowerPoint presentation to depict the modes of transmission of infections and ways to prevent outbreaks. For proper hand-washing techniques, use a "glow light" to test for thorough cleaning. The Centers for Disease Control and Prevention website is a good resource for teaching tools (http://www.cdc.gov). If your community has an Infection Control director, have that individual present this portion of the program.

REDUCING RETURN-TO-HOSPITAL RATES

Currently, one of the main focuses within long-term care is reducing a community's return-to-hospital rate. Due in large part to passage in 2010 of the Patient Protection and Affordable Care Act, healthcare reform laws are affecting what payments hospitals receive for services rendered. It behooves a community to do everything possible to make sure residents are receiving optimal care in order to reduce the need for hospital admission and to keep residents in the Neighborhood. One way to achieve this is by training new team members to thoroughly assess residents, which includes getting to know them well, a basic principle of person-centered care. By knowing a resident's baseline, caregivers are more apt to notice subtle changes that can lead to serious consequences. Paying close attention to variations in hydration status, decreases or increases in weight, difficulty with ambulation, skin temperature changes, changes in mental status, slurred speech, lethargy, and any other departure from a resident's normal state will help the resident stay healthier and possibly reduce the need to go to a hospital. Hospital stays can be devastating to an older adult.

When at all possible, it is best to treat residents at the community. The resident physician or nurse practitioner can order tests as necessary, such as labs to rule out urinary tract infections. Portable X-rays can be done on site for suspicion of pneumonia. Even with these interventions, sometimes hospital stays are unavoidable. These times can be very upsetting and traumatic for residents and their families. When a resident is sent to the hospital, he or she often experiences additional problems, such as confusion in response to being in a strange environment with different caregivers as well as an increased risk of developing pressure ulcers and hospital-acquired infections. Remind new team members to be aware of the stress and anxiety an unexpected hospital stay can have on residents and their loved ones.

If your community has specific tools or programs for assessing residents or recommended procedures to explain pathways of care, be sure to include them in the orientation program. If possible, have a physician or nurse practitioner present this segment in order to provide in-depth details about the effects of illness on the geriatric population.

EVALUATIONS

Every orientation process should include an evaluation tool to critique the program and make changes as needed. It is important to solicit the opinions of the new team members because the orientation program is their first taste of your community and will have the longest lasting impression. You want to make sure you are doing everything possible to address their needs and equip them with the proper tools to perform their jobs to the best of their abilities. Evaluations should be done immediately after the orientation classes are concluded and again after 30 to 60 days of working in the Neighborhood. Chapter 11 discusses evaluations in further detail and provides examples of evaluation forms to use.

SUMMARY

Using these 12 components as the core of your orientation will form the basis of a thorough and effective program. While this list may appear daunting, keep in mind that the goal is to provide a general introduction to the community and its policies and procedures. Be creative in the way each topic is presented by balancing lecture with videos, interchanging speakers, and allowing the orientees to participate. This will keep the program effective without becoming overwhelming for both you and the new team members you are training.

Establish the Needs of Your Community
REVIEW

- Identify the needs and goals of the community.

- Give an overview of the Nursing department.

- Identify service providers and demonstrate how products are used with residents.

- Describe the culture of the community and person-centered care practices.

- Provide in-depth electronic medical records training for all levels of care-givers.

- Conduct Alzheimer's and dementia training for all new staff.

- Clearly define the community's policy on preventing resident abuse and neglect and maintaining resident dignity.

- Outline procedures for accidents and injuries as they relate to residents, staff, and guests.

- Test the skills of all new team members according to discipline.

- Provide detailed admission and discharge instructions.

- Explain the policy regarding infection control and require new team members to demonstrate proper procedures.

- Discuss the community's efforts to reduce return-to-hospital rates.

- Gather feedback on the orientation program from orientees to enhance and improve future classes.

NOTES

_____

_____

_____

_____

_____

_____

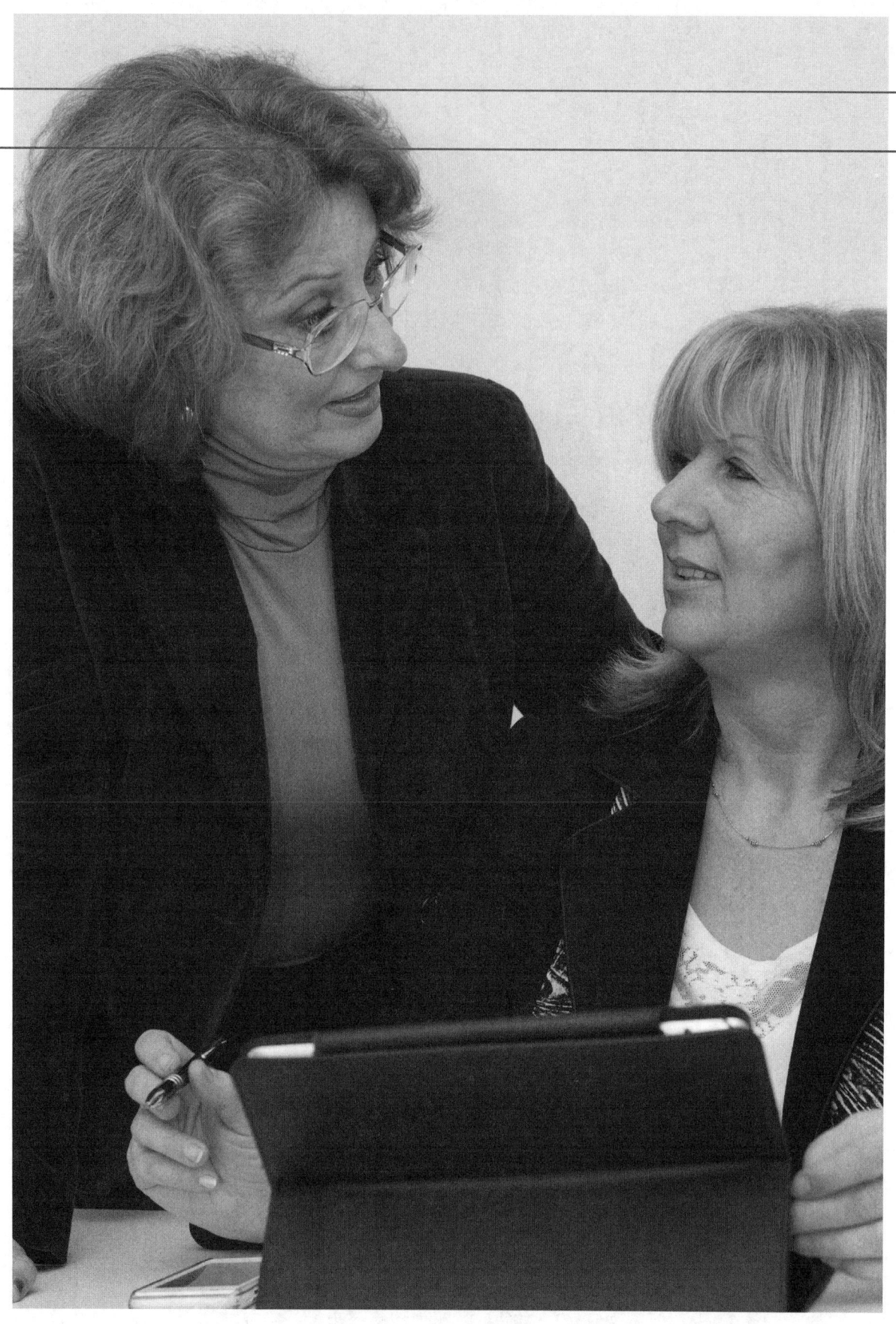

CHAPTER 2

Creating an Agenda

Once you have chosen the topics to be presented as part of the orientation program, the next step is to create an agenda, which will outline exactly what you will be covering and give the orientees an idea of what to expect. The agenda should be broken down into manageable segments as well as include the approximate time frames to cover each section and the name and title of each presenter.

The agenda items will vary depending on the type of employees being trained and the different programs your organization offers. When creating an agenda, follow these guidelines:

1. Allow enough time to adequately present each topic. Consider that the orientation program is an introduction to your community and take care not to overwhelm new hires with too much information. Touch on important topics without delving too deeply into the subject matter. The mentors will pick up where you left off when there is ample time for one-on-one training in the Neighborhood or Household (Chapter 3).

2. Incorporate time for breaks and lunch, and announce at the beginning of the program approximately when each break will occur. Also, direct staff to the restrooms and, if applicable, smoking areas.

3. Rehearse the topics to determine the length of time to cover each one and include time for conversation and discussion. Make sure each presenter is well versed on the subject matter and has the necessary knowledge to answer questions from the group.

4. Allow the orientees ample time to participate in the training when completing return demonstrations or skills testing (Chapter 6). They should not feel rushed or hurried.

5. Include time to sign and complete any necessary forms or pa-

perwork. Review each document to ensure it is completed accurately and legibly.

6. Prioritize the information by devoting more time to the most important topics.

7. Review the list of topics with the leaders in your community to ensure you have developed a comprehensive program that meets the needs of the community. Invite input from department managers based on the areas of concern they feel new team members need more thorough education on.

8. Collaborate with the Human Resources and Nursing department leaders to ensure your organizational requirements are addressed in the orientation program. Review your policies and procedures and determine which are necessary to include and emphasize.

9. Include any subjects that are required according to local, state, and federal guidelines. This can include, for example, immunization requirements as mandated in accordance with your geographic area.

10. If videos are included in your agenda, intersperse them periodically throughout the entire orientation program. It is advisable to pause the videos from time to time in order to allow for discussion and interaction and to help maintain the attention of the group. Allow time for orientees to offer comments and share past experiences, which will promote a sense of involvement. Hearing that your co-workers have experienced similar situations and learning how they dealt with them expands one's knowledge base and creates bonds within the group. It also builds relationships that will extend beyond the orientation and mentoring period.

Once you finalize the list of topics, organize the agenda by discipline. For example, all participants (CNAs, CMTs, RNs, and LPNs) attend the first day because the information universally applies to every staff member. The training for CNAs is completed after day one. The remainder of the group continues on through the morning of day two, at which time the CMT portion is completed. The afternoon of the second day pertains to nurses only. This agenda fulfills everyone's needs and avoids having staff attend classes that do not pertain to them. The sample Nursing Department Orientation Program Agenda at the end of the chapter is typical for a 2-day orientation.

In addition to the agenda, create a manual or binder with tabbed sections for each orientee to take notes and keep as a resource. Number each topic on the agenda to correspond directly with its tabbed section in the binder. Insert copies of PowerPoint presentations, handouts, informational and reference sheets, and so forth in the appropriate-tabbed sections. Prepare a binder for each orientee with his or her photo ID and badge holder. Place the binders around the table to be used for the training or on desks before the new team members arrive. You may also choose to include a pen with your community name and logo with each binder. These are all ways to show you are serious about investing your time, effort, and resources to ensure each new team member will be successful in his or her position. It also creates an immediate sense of caring and appreciation for the talent and skills each individual brings to your community.

Organize the contents of each binder by discipline according to the information that is pertinent to each scope of practice. This means you will have separate binders for CNAs, CMTs, and nurses. For example, the information for the CNA will be limited to the first nine sections of the agenda. CMTs will be given information up to and including section 15, and nurses will receive the largest binder with every section included. For the CNA content, you may choose to use a small pocket folder instead of a binder since their packets will contain less paperwork.

When compiling a folder or binder of information to give to the orientees, include any forms or paperwork that are required to be signed at the time of hire. Place these forms in a separate section of the binder or pocket in the folder so they are easy to access. Make duplicates so new hires have copies of the important policies and agreements they have signed. Signature pages may include the following:

- electronic signature contract for protecting electronic medical records (see the sample Privacy and Protected Information Compliance Form at the end of the chapter)
- HIPAA agreement
- attendance and absenteeism guidelines
- vacation, sick days, and paid time off guidelines
- disciplinary guidelines (verbal warnings, written warnings, final warnings)
- acknowledgment of receiving the employee handbook
- immunization verifications
- checklist of each item presented during the orientation with signature page acknowledging the topics that were taught (see the sample Nursing Orientation Program Checklist at the end of the chapter)

Inform the new hires in advance of what to expect during the orientation process so they can arrive prepared. Let them know the hours they will be expected to be present since they may vary from their regularly scheduled shifts. Inform them if lunch and snacks will be provided or if they need to bring their own. Advise them to be well rested and prepared for a full session of learning. Sometimes new staff members are still working another job during orientation. It is unreasonable to expect that a nurse who just worked the night shift will come to your orientation class awake, alert, and able to absorb the information you are presenting. It does not bode well for an orientee to be falling asleep during lecture or videos. Outlining the orientation expectations in advance will give new staff the opportunity to be able to put their best foot forward and be successful.

By making a good first impression in preparing the orientation program materials, your new team members will feel appreciated and comfortable in the community. Their level of excitement to begin a new career will be heightened as they anticipate a long-term relationship with your organization.

Creating an Agenda

REVIEW

- Make a good first impression by welcoming new staff and expending time and resources to ensure their success.

- Create a comprehensive agenda.

- Stagger the agenda according to discipline.

- Prepare a binder or manual for new staff to take notes and keep as a reference.

- Include required signature pages in the binder.

- Define for the new team members the orientation expectations prior to class.

NOTES

_____

_____

_____

_____

_____

_____

_____

_____

_____

_____

Nursing Department Orientation Program Agenda

DAY 1 (ALL STAFF)

TIME	TOPIC
8:00–8:20	Introductions/Overview of Nursing Department
8:20–9:00	Dignity and Confidentiality Issues
9:00–9:30	Abuse and Neglect in the Elderly
9:30–10:15	Infection Control in Long-Term Care
	10-minute break
10:25–11:00	Safe Transfer and Lifting
11:00–11:30	Tour of Community
11:30–12:00	Lunch
12:00–12:30	Product Information (Skin, Wound, and Incontinence Care)
12:30–1:15	Reduce Return-to-Hospital Rate
	10-minute break
1:25–2:30	Electronic Medical Records and Passwords
2:30–3:30	Activities of Daily Living Documentation

DAY 2 A.M. (RN, LPN, CMT)

TIME	TOPIC
8:00–8:45	Adjunct Services (Lab/Radiology/Pharmacy)
8:45–9:15	Physical Therapy Services and Documentation
9:15–10:00	Medication Administration/Destruction/Documentation
	10-minute break
10:10–10:30	Nebulizer Treatments
10:30–11:00	Blood Glucose Monitoring and Insulin Administration
11:00–11:45	Medication Knowledge Test
11:45–12:15	Lunch

DAY 2 P.M. (RN, LPN)

TIME	TOPIC
12:45–1:45	Admission Process
1:45–2:00	Order Entry
2:00–2:30	Accidents and Injuries
	10-minute break
2:30–3:00	Wound Care (Assessment and Documentation)
3:00–3:30	Progress Notes
3:30–4:00	End-of-Life Care

Nursing Orientation Program Checklist

NAME _____

DEPARTMENT _____

TITLE _____ DATE OF HIRE _____

The following topics were reviewed during orientation:

☑ **Departmental Education**
Parking
Clocking in/out
Dress code and personal hygiene
Pay periods/Holidays/Personal time
Hours of work by shift
Call-in process

☑ **Products and Services**
Skin and wound care products
Incontinence care products
Safety products (syringes, sharps, containers)

☑ **Culture Change and Person-Centered Care**
Definition and structure of a Neighborhood
My role in a person-centered Neighborhood
Teamwork
Building relationships with residents and families

☑ **Electronic Medical Records Training**
How to log in/out
Data entry
Email
Passwords

☑ **Alzheimer's and Dementia Training**

☑ **Abuse and Neglect and Resident Dignity**
Upholding HIPAA regulations
Respecting residents' rights

☑ **Accidents and Injuries**
How to report
How to document

☑ **Skills Testing (per discipline)**
CNA skills
CMT skills
Nurse skills

☑ **Admission and Discharge Process**
New resident admission
Re-admission of resident returning from hospital
Resident discharge to hospital or home
Resident death

☑ **Infection Control**
Hand-washing
Blood-borne pathogens
Isolation

☑ **Reducing Return-to-Hospital Rates**
Assessing residents
Reporting changes from normal status
Following paths to care

☑ **Evaluations**

I confirm that the Nursing Orientation Program covered the topics listed above and that I have a full understanding of the subjects presented.

_____   _____
Orientee   Date

I certify that the above-named employee successfully completed the Nursing Orientation Program.

_____   _____
Instructor   Date

Privacy and Protected Information Compliance Form

NAME _____

DEPARTMENT _____

TITLE _____ DATE OF HIRE _____

I have been trained on the policy and procedure regarding the Health Insurance Portability and Accountability Act of 1996 (HIPAA) and how it relates to my specific job description. I fully understand that I have an obligation to take all necessary measures to protect and maintain the highest level of privacy regarding resident information, including personal, medical, and confidential information.

I agree to use any private resident information for the sole purpose of performing my specific assigned job duties.

I acknowledge that any information related to residents must be kept private at all times, including while I am not at work.

I agree not to use any reference to a resident on all forms of social media.

I will keep all passwords confidential and will take all necessary precautions to keep electronic health information secure by:

     a. Not disclosing my password to anyone

     b. Not allowing other staff to chart under my name or password

     c. Closing all computer screens containing resident information upon completion of charting

I also understand and agree that failure to comply with the policy and procedure regarding HIPAA will result in my being subject to appropriate disciplinary action, up to and including termination.

_____   _____
Orientee   Date

_____   _____
Instructor   Date

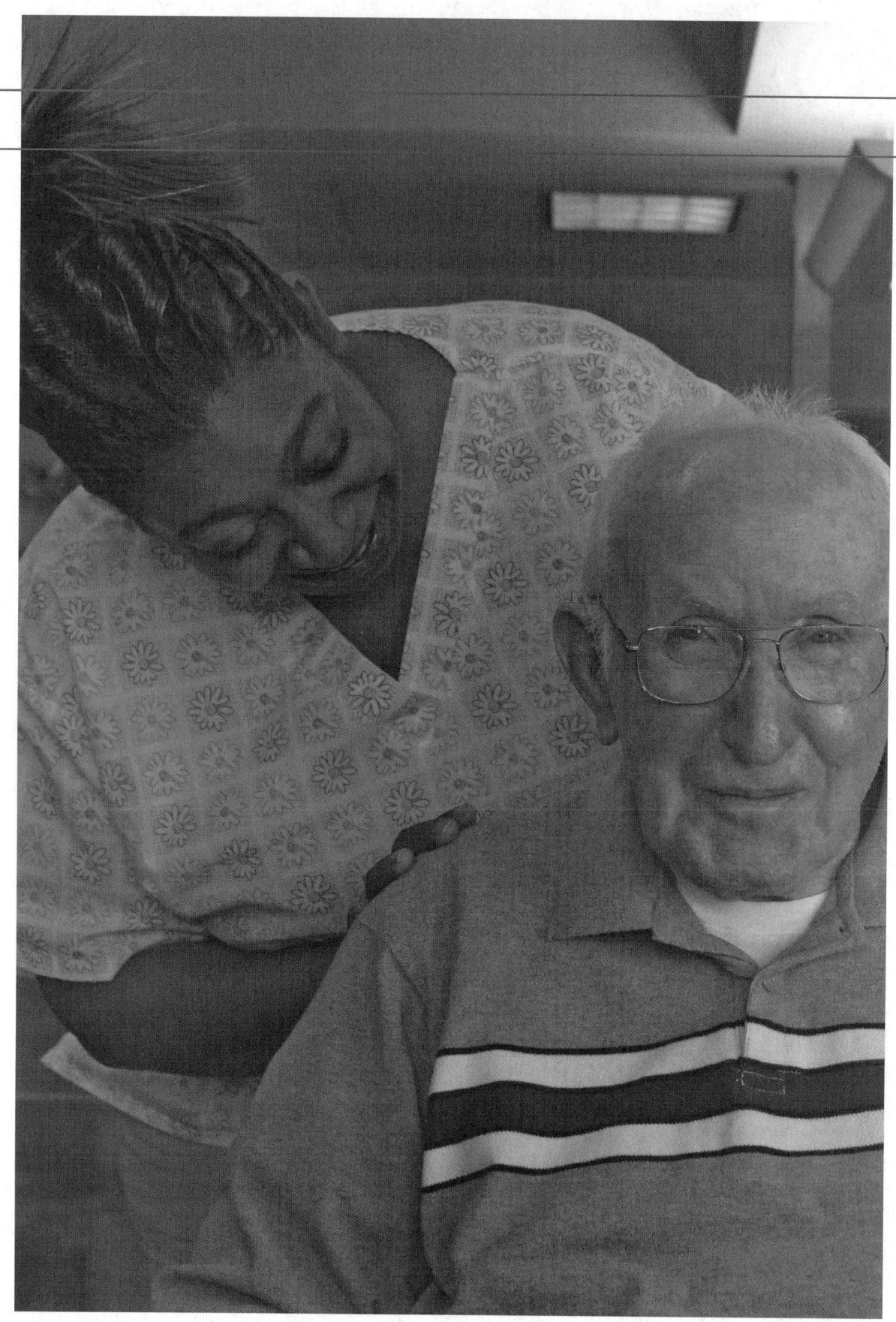

CHAPTER 3

Establishing a Mentor Training Program

Conducting an orientation program is only one half of educating new team members. The second half is to pair them each with a good mentor who will continue the education process. Mentors are trained staff who are dedicated to helping new team members transition from "new employees" to productive, contributing co-workers. Mentors serve as peers in the Neighborhood and perform many roles for new hires, including the following:

- provide education, guidance, support, and encouragement
- assist new team members to develop and enhance problem-solving skills
- encourage independence and good decision-making abilities
- help orientees transition into the community at large
- ensure orientees successfully demonstrate all skills
- provide feedback to supervisors about orientees' performance
- help orientees set goals and assist them in achieving those goals
- encourage orientees to find ways to utilize their strengths and assist in addressing their weaknesses

This list is a tall order for any one staff member; therefore, it is important to seek out the right people for the task. There are those employees we often wish we could "clone" or had five more of just like them; they are the ones who would be great mentors. However, even the best nurse or nurse's aide may not be a good teacher. Teaching requires excellent communication skills, patience, and the willingness to help others succeed. It takes a huge commitment of time and resources, which makes it essential that the mentor be organized, timely, and thorough in his or her duties. Mentors must work well independently and possess strong critical thinking skills. Additionally, they must demonstrate excellent technique to the orientees during training to ensure new team members demonstrate the required skills to complete their tasks.

Becoming a mentor has many positive aspects for those who choose to serve in this very important role in your community. Mentors build their skills and gain a higher level of confidence as they see the impact they have on new team members. Mentoring programs help develop and promote leaders within your organization who have a vested interest in providing quality care to residents. Mentors serve as role models for others to apply themselves, excel in their positions, and advance their careers. Mentoring also increases employee retention and reduces undue stress on new and existing staff, which ultimately saves time and money. Overall, mentoring is a person-centered approach that benefits everyone involved.

To start a mentor program in your community, have interested staff complete and submit an application. They must also have a written recommendation from their direct supervisor since they are the ones who are most familiar with the applicant's work history. The supervisors should understand that an applicant might be denied acceptance into the mentor program based on his or her prior performance, attendance, work ethic, attitude, and ability to work well with other members of the team. Encourage supervisors to share constructive criticism about applicants and to be fair in determining which staff will orient new team members because the mentors will have a direct effect on their performance outcomes.

Mentors should also have enthusiasm and a strong desire to teach others. Select staff from each discipline and, if possible, from each shift. The orientees begin working alongside their mentor immediately after the orientation program. Each new team member begins on the day shift for the first few weeks since that is when there are more opportunities to witness a greater variety of admissions, discharges, delivery and processing of medications, lab draws, physical therapy sessions, and so forth. It is also the time when new staff can interact with other departments, such as Payroll and Human Resources. After the first few weeks on the day shift, the new team members will continue their training with mentors on their respective regularly scheduled shifts. At the end of the chapter, see the sample Mentor Application Form and Supervisor Recommendation Form for Mentor Program, which can be used in seeking out prospective mentors.

Once a group of mentors has been selected, you can begin training them. In welcoming everyone to the mentor training program, begin by acknowledging their decision to become mentors and praise them for choosing to make a difference. Emphasize the following:

- They have been selected by their supervisors because they have a proven track record of reliability, dependability, and excellent skills.
- They will sign a mentor agreement and agree to abide by the expectations listed therein (see sample Mentor Agreement at the end of the chapter).
- They will train new team members to adopt the same qualities and work ethic they themselves possess.
- They will have a direct impact on the success of the orientees.
- Their mentoring will help others understand person-centered care and enhance the living experience of residents.
- They will be instrumental in assisting to build a team of dedicated employees for the community.

Provide an agenda showing the topics that will be covered during the mentor training (see the sample Mentor Training Agenda at the end of the chapter, including brief descriptions of each section to be covered). Ensure all applicants are fully aware of the commitment they are expected to make from the start. If any applicant is having second thoughts, now is the time to find out so no one's time is wasted. Each prospective mentor must be willing to uphold the mission statement of your community and act accordingly as a representative of the organization as a whole.

It is very important to have consistency by assigning each new team member to only one mentor. Each mentor has his or her own routine and style of teaching, and there are too many inconsistencies in training when staff members are shuffled from one mentor to another throughout the course of the orientation process. When making assignments, the new team member will work the same shift as his or her mentor, even if it will not ultimately be a regular shift assignment. Encourage mentors to express early on in the training process if they feel they are not a suitable fit for their assigned new team member and make changes as soon as possible.

Lengths of assignments will vary based on each new hire's experience and level of expertise. The mentor will confer with the new team member's supervisor and make recommendations on when he or she is ready to work independently. To prevent burnout, nursing supervisors should be aware of how often and for how long each mentor trains new team members. Supervisors should periodically ask mentors if they need to take a break for a few weeks. This will help keep them from becoming too overwhelmed and perhaps deciding to quit the mentor program.

The mentors should receive compensation for their time and efforts. There are several ways to remunerate your mentors. One method is to pay an increased hourly wage during the shifts when they are working as mentors. One of the drawbacks to this approach is that it may be difficult to track the exact number of hours or days when mentoring actually occurred. Another method is a tiered compensation plan, which is more comprehensive and attractive to mentors. A flat rate for each new team member who is mentored is paid in stages throughout the entire orientation process (see the sample Tiered Compensation Plan for Mentors at the end of the chapter).

The mentor, new team member, and nursing administration each benefit from a tiered compensation package for several reasons, including:

- acts as an incentive to attract new mentors
- encourages mentors to perform their duties and responsibilities in a timely manner
- promotes continuous training beyond the initial 30 to 90 days of orientation
- inspires new team members to stay focused and become proficient in their new roles
- improves employee retention and reduces turnover rates
- reinforces a person-centered care approach
- maintains consistent staffing to provide better resident outcomes

The nursing supervisor will ensure the requirements for each tier have been fulfilled and will authorize the appropriate payment for the mentor.

Inspire new mentors to be successful in their new role by encouraging them to create a list of goals to remember as they work with new team members, including the following:

- We were once all new to the team ourselves—try to remember how that felt and be kind and understanding in addressing the orientees' needs.
- Being the new kid on the block is like traveling to a foreign country where you don't speak the language. Give new team members time to comprehend new concepts and procedures, and expect that it will take several times to learn them all and do them right.
- Remember that although you may be teaching them only one thing at the moment, they are trying to learn many new tasks, which can be overwhelming.

- The best teachers are those who already have experience acting in certain roles and dealing with specific situations they are trying to teach others about. Use your experience as a resource to help anticipate any barriers to learning that orientees may be trying to overcome, such as being a new nurse, feeling insecure in his or her skill level, or feeling out of place in a new environment. If you feel you need help in teaching a particular portion or segment of the orientation, ask a fellow colleague for his or her advice or expertise. A mentor should never guess at responses or make up answers in responding to questions from new team members.

- Applaud the accomplishments of the orientees, no matter how small. A little praise goes a long way to boost their spirits and reinforce their commitment to excel.

Hold mentor meetings to bring the group together and discuss both the positive and negative aspects of their work in guiding new team members. This is a good way to exchange ideas and teaching methods. If there is an outstanding mentor, you may wish to appoint that person as the lead and have him or her schedule and run the meetings.

Periodic training for mentors should occur at least every 4–6 months. Poll the group to identify the educational needs they may have and deliver in-service trainings to meet those needs. If necessary, bring in outside resources, such as the pharmacist or a nurse practitioner, to present a training session.

Supervisors should periodically evaluate mentors to ensure they are meeting the expectations of their role in introducing new team members to the Neighborhood. Feedback from the orientees taken from the evaluations and interviews they complete as part of the training program will help determine if they have been properly educated to perform their jobs well (see Chapter 11). Observing mentors and orientees during the mentoring process is a good way to rate the effectiveness of a mentor's communication skills. For example, observe a mentor teaching an orientee a skill such as cleaning a foley catheter bag. Carefully watch the exchange of information, then observe the orientee performing the task independently to see if he or she fully comprehended the concept by showing an accurate return demonstration. If the supervisor feels the mentor has achieved or surpassed the goals in training new hires, then the evaluation can substantiate a pay increase for the mentor.

A solid mentor program is an important component to the success of the orientation program. Empower your team members to strive to reach their full potential as well as to help others reach theirs.

Establishing a Mentor Training Program
REVIEW

- Mentors are essential to the orientation program in introducing new team members to the Neighborhood.

- Mentors must complete an application form and obtain their supervisor's recommendation.

- Select mentors based on performance history, reliability, and work ethic.

- Mentors sign an agreement and abide by its terms.

- Evaluate and train mentors prior to having them work with new hires.

- Create a skills demonstration checklist for each discipline to be used by the mentors in evaluating new team members.

- Compensate mentors for their work.

- Provide mentors with continuing education.

- Elect a lead mentor and encourage the group to meet regularly to discuss their work in guiding new team members.

NOTES

_____

_____

_____

_____

_____

_____

_____

Mentor Agreement

I, _____, agree to be a
mentor to new team members. As a mentor, I will:

- be committed to upholding the mission statement of the community

- assist new team members in becoming skilled and competent in their roles

- report to my supervisor any concerns that I may have regarding a new team member

- complete all necessary paperwork and training with new team members according to schedule

- use my knowledge and experience when training new team members and utilize the orientation checklist as a guideline for training

- understand that I will participate in ongoing in-services and trainings to stay current on new policies and procedures

- understand that if I am not meeting the expectations of the role of mentor, I may be relieved of my duties as a mentor

_____   _____
Mentor's Signature   Date

_____   _____
Supervisor's Signature   Date

Mentor Application Form

NAME _____

DATE OF HIRE _____

CURRENT POSITION _____ LENGTH OF TIME _____

PREVIOUS POSITION (if applicable) _____

Please answer the following questions:

1. What strengths do you possess that would be beneficial to your role as a mentor?

   _____

   _____

   _____

2. Identify the top three challenges new team members face:

   a. _____

   b. _____

   c. _____

3. Describe how you would help new team members overcome these challenges:

   _____

   _____

   _____

4. Describe your teaching style:

   _____

   _____

   _____

continued

Mentor Application Form *cont.*

NAME _____

5. Explain why you would like to become a mentor:

    _____

    _____

    _____

6. What are your goals as a mentor and how do you hope to achieve them?

    _____

    _____

    _____

Mentor Training Agenda

DATE _____

TIME _____

LOCATION _____

SECTION	TITLE	DESCRIPTION
1	Introductions	Meet your fellow mentors
2	Job description	Detailed list of topics the mentor is expected to review with each orientee during the orientation process
3	Mentor Agreement	Agreement to be signed by each mentor confirming his or her commitment to the Mentor Program
4	Skills competency verification	Mentors will demonstrate knowledge and competence in skills they are expected to teach to orientees
5	Skills demonstration checklist	Checklist mentors will complete, sign, and date when an orientee has demonstrated the knowledge and competence related to his or her respective discipline
6	Timeliness of paperwork	Schedule detailing the timeline for submitting completed paperwork
7	Learning styles and personalities	Recognizing and understanding varied personalities and styles of learning and how to relate to them
8	Additional training	Ongoing training sessions for mentors to enhance their skill sets and to learn new ways to teach new team members
9	Characteristics of a good mentor	Qualities every good mentor must possess

continued

Enhancing Staff Retention in Person-Centered Care Environments for Older Adults: How to Create and Implement a Comprehensive Orientation Program, by Janine M. Lange. Copyright © 2016 by Health Professions Press, Inc. All rights reserved. www.healthpropress.com.

Mentor Training Agenda *cont.*

1. *Introductions:* Have the mentors introduce themselves and state the reasons why they have chosen to become mentors and their goals for the mentoring program.

2. *Job description:* Provide a comprehensive list of all of the duties mentors will be expected to perform while guiding new staff, including becoming oriented to the Neighborhood, teaching policies and procedures, assessing skills, completing orientation checklists, submitting completed paperwork, etc.

3. *Mentor Agreement:* Have each mentor read and sign the Mentor Agreement. Provide a signed copy for them to keep for their records.

4. *Skills competency verification:* Review the skills each mentor will be required to observe according to discipline and the process for verifying an orientee's competency through either written exam or return demonstration.

5. *Skills demonstration checklist:* Provide a copy of the skills demonstration checklist used to verify the skills of orientees. Test skills related to each discipline. Ensure the mentors understand each task on the checklist. The mentor will observe each skill and document whether the orientee performed each one within expectations or whether the orientee needs additional training. Create the checklist based on the services offered by your community and the guidelines for each individual disciplines' scope of practice. Abide by your local, state, and federal regulations as well as the policies and procedures of your community.

6. *Timeliness of paperwork:* Provide a timeline detailing when completed paperwork is due in order to receive compensation for mentoring. Define the consequences if paperwork is incomplete or late.

7. *Learning styles and personalities:* Describe the varied adult learning styles and personalities the mentors will encounter in working with orientees and provide suggestions on ways to train and teach. Let the mentors know that not everyone can adapt to another person's style of learning or teaching and it is perfectly acceptable for an orientee to request a different mentor. Reinforce the fact that if this does occur, it is not necessarily a reflection of the mentor's skills or talent.

8. *Additional training:* Provide a calendar with scheduled dates for ongoing training classes and emphasize that mentors are expected to make a commitment to attend each session. Encourage mentors to make suggestions for training they would like to participate in or feel they need.

9. *Characteristics of a good mentor:* Describe the qualities that a good mentor possesses, such as the following:
   - assumes responsibility for imparting knowledge and skills to orientees
   - demonstrates a positive attitude and admirable behavior
   - possesses excellent communication skills
   - committed to upholding and exemplifying the mission statement of the organization
   - serves as a resource for information, encouragement, and inspiration
   - sets professional and personal goals and strives to achieve them
   - places a high value on continuing education

Supervisor Recommendation Form for Mentor Program

To be considered for the mentoring program, each applicant must meet the following requirements:

- No more than three absences within the past 12 months

- No tardies or late arrivals

- Annual performance review with "Meets" or "Exceeds Expectations" for prior year

- No verbal or written warnings within the past 24 months

Please confirm the applicant's qualifications and provide your feedback below:

_____

_____

_____

As the direct supervisor for _____, I

☐   recommend the applicant for the Mentor Program

☐   do not recommend the applicant for the Mentor Program

_____   _____
Supervisor's Signature   Date

Tiered Compensation Plan for Mentors

TIER	DESCRIPTION	MENTOR PAY
1	• New team member is mentored on the Neighborhood • Skills checklist completed and submitted within 30 days of new team member working on the Neighborhood	$25.00
2	• New team member completes 90-day probationary period • New team member demonstrates all skills accurately • New team member is hired permanently	$50.00
3	• New team member completes 1 year of employment • New team member's job performance is evaluated as acceptable and with no deficiencies	$50.00

Dollar amounts represent a one-time fee paid to the mentor for each mentee.

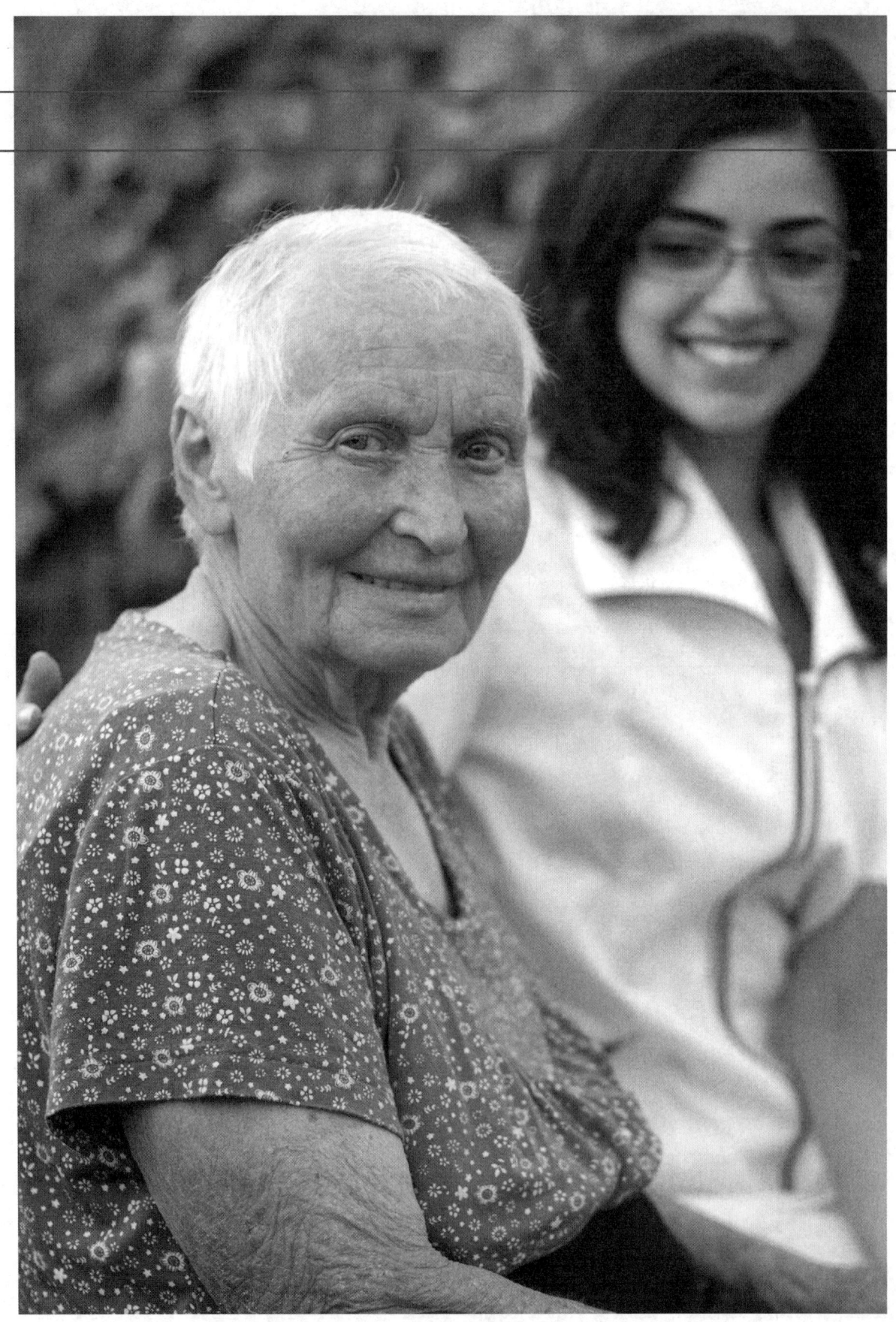

CHAPTER 4

Defining the Culture of Your Community

Although the concepts of culture change and person-centered care are not new in long-term care, they may be new to staff who are joining your community. Since there are many varying interpretations of person-centered care, your community's approach may be different from others'. To begin educating new hires on the culture of your community, ask the class to define *person-centered care* and to describe what it means to each of them. Some new team members have either never heard of the concept or never worked in a culture-change environment, while others may be quite familiar with the practices. Either way, it is important to portray an accurate picture of exactly what culture change and person-centered care look like in your community.

Person-centered care is based on the core values of personhood, dignity, respect, and personal choices. It honors each individual's right to decide how he or she wants to be cared for and allows for accommodations to meet his or her needs. For example, in your own home no one tells you when to wake up, take your medications, eat your meals, or shower, so why is it acceptable to force these rules and restrictions on residents of a long- or short-term care community? Culture change allows residents to live meaningful, purposeful, and enriching lives to the best of their capabilities.

Familiarize new team members with the titles, terminology, and language your community prefers in support of person-centered care practices. Many aspects of person-centered care appear and sound different and thus the nomenclature of a culture change environment differs from typical care settings. For example, instead of *diaper*, the word *brief* is used. A person once referred to as a "feeder" is now known as "one who needs dining assistance." Those receiving care are referred to as *resident* or *guest* as opposed to *patient*. What were once called *units* are now referred to as *Neighborhoods* or *Households*. Staff also have different titles, such as *care companion* versus *certified nurse aide*, *team leader* versus *assistant director of nursing*, and *Neighborhood nurse* versus *charge nurse*.

Care given to residents in a person-centered community relies greatly on the relationships formed between staff and residents. Staff are encouraged to learn as much as possible about those they are caring for on a daily basis and to familiarize themselves with their habits and preferences. For example, knowing that a resident loved to garden opens up many opportunities to engage in meaningful conversations. This is especially useful if a resident becomes agitated or upset during daily care, such as bathing. By talking about topics of interest with a resident, caregivers can focus the resident's attention on something he or she enjoys rather than the task at hand.

Also discuss with new hires how your community creates a home-like environment for residents, even in cases where physical changes to the environment are not structurally or monetarily feasible. Neighborhoods or Households are decorated and furnished to appeal to those who reside there. Paint, wallpaper, and window dressings are more personalized and inviting and less institutional. Chairs and furniture create comfortable areas for residents to relax in or to sit and read a book or magazine. Fireplaces add a soft, warm atmosphere reminiscent of home. Many Neighborhoods have their own kitchens and dining rooms. The scent of food being prepared enhances the dining experience and entices appetites, which helps reduce unplanned weight loss. Overhead paging, call light bells, and the loud disruptive noises of utility carts are significantly reduced or eliminated completely when possible. Staff can carry pagers that vibrate to alert them when a resident needs assistance. Laundry rooms on Neighborhoods offer many benefits, including that laundry is less likely to become lost, and residents can assist in folding laundry to encourage participation and purpose in the daily activities of life. As you tour the community with new team members, point out the differences in contrast to a typical long-term care setting.

Educate new team members on the daily operations of each Neighborhood and provide a clear set of expectations and job duties. Some person-centered care approaches that may be new to orientees include the following:

- allowing staff to sit and eat meals with residents to encourage conversation and increased consumption
- team members engaging in one-on-one or group activities with residents, such as reading the newspaper together
- using residents' preferred personal care items, such as shower gels and body lotions, instead of those supplied by the community

- adjusting medication times to accommodate residents who sleep late, retire early, or choose not to wait to eat after receiving their medicine

The responsibilities of Neighborhood teams, or *families*, can also vary. For example, nursing staff and homemakers have different duties within the Household. Care companions attend to residents' physical needs and activities of daily living, while homemakers prepare and serve meals and maintain the cleanliness of the Neighborhood. Although they each have distinct duties, it is imperative that team members work together to provide excellent care for residents.

You will also need to define the hierarchy in your community and introduce the key leaders, such as clinical team leaders and Neighborhood team leaders. Keep in mind that the titles of staff may be unfamiliar to new team members and they may need a little time to remember names and duties. Use a schematic, such as the following, to help them grasp the structure of the Neighborhood team members. Change the titles to suit your community.

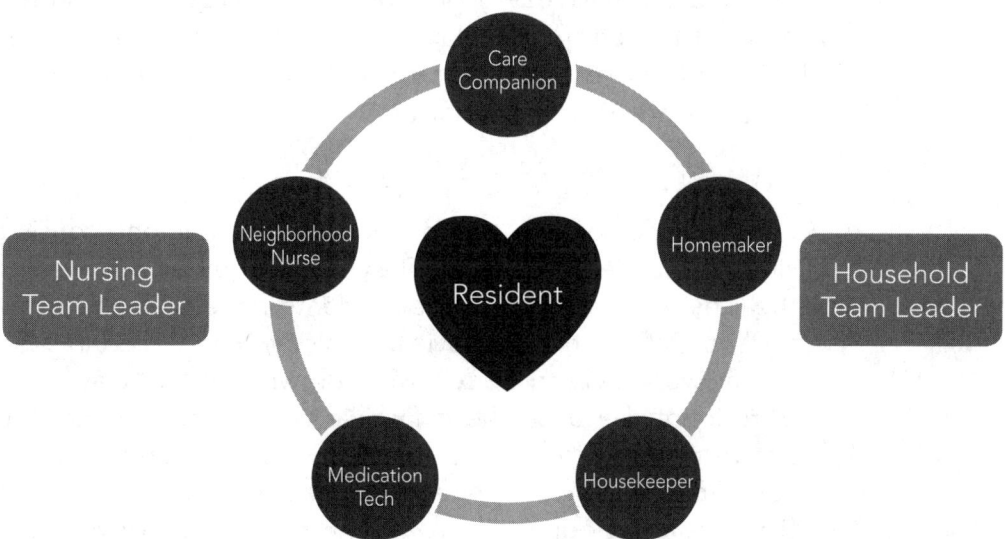

The nursing team leader oversees the Neighborhood nursing staff, including care companions (CNAs), certified medication technicians (CMTs), and nurses. The leaders ensure nursing staff follow policies and procedures, including with respect to medication administration and documentation, infection control, attendance and punctuality, continuing education, HIPAA laws, and so forth. The Household team leader supervises the housekeepers and homemakers, ensuring the Neighborhood is kept clean and orderly and the meals are properly prepared in accordance with all federal, state, and local requirements.

Stress to new team members how the Neighborhood team works together to maintain the highest level of care for residents, around whom everything revolves. For example, in the event one team member is overwhelmed, the expectation is that other members of the Household will lend a hand in order to complete necessary tasks. In this setting, there is no room for staff to quibble over who is doing more work on any given day; it is about how the cumulative efforts of the team meet the needs of residents. If a care companion has several baths on a particular morning, the nurse should step in and help provide dining assistance to residents who require help with breakfast. A homemaker is qualified to sit and read with a resident or play a game of cards or checkers when he or she notices a resident becomes agitated, bored, or confused or is experiencing the effects of sundowning (a state of confusion at the end of the day and into the night characterized by anxiety, aggression, or ignoring directions as well as pacing or wandering). Nurse and Household leaders can walk with a resident who tends to wander to reduce the risk of flight.

Ultimately, with every member of the Neighborhood team working in unison throughout the day, the workload is actually lessened. The following is an example to share with new team members to help them grasp the concept of teamwork.

Mary and Allison are two of the care companions consistently assigned to a Neighborhood. They work together very well and know the likes and dislikes of all the residents in the Household. Mary cares for Mrs. Brown and Mr. Davies. This day, Mary called in sick and was not at work. Allison added Mrs. Brown and Mr. Davies to her list of residents because she is familiar with them and knows that Mrs. Brown needs a lot of encouragement at mealtimes. She has been consistently losing weight and is very weak. Allison notices that Mrs. Brown is upset during breakfast and not eating or even drinking because Mary is not there to assist her. Rather than ignore the situation, Allison moves to Mrs. Brown's side of the table and encourages her to eat. She has to continually bring the glass of orange juice to Mrs. Brown's mouth to help her drink. Allison does not want to neglect the other residents in her care, so she lets the nurse leader know her concerns and enlists her assistance. Realizing Allison's concerns, the nurse leader restructures her duties to make herself available to help with the other residents while Allison continues to assist Mrs. Brown. Everyone was fed and no resident was left unattended. Had the team not worked together, the outcome could have been very different. If no one had aided Mrs. Brown, she would probably have not eaten breakfast or had anything to drink. Being frail and weak already, the lack of food or beverage could have led to complications such as dehydration or confusion, which could have caused Mrs. Brown to become disoriented and increase her risk of falling. A fall could have terrible consequences, such as a broken hip, which would have sent Mrs. Brown to the hospital. This worse-case scenario was thankfully avoided due to the concerted efforts of the Neighborhood team.

To a resident, not seeing the care companion he or she is accustomed to on a certain day can be very troubling and upsetting. It is important for new team members to understand that what may appear to be a small, insignificant change to them can have profound effects on a resident. Good communication skills, teamwork, and close relationships with residents help the Neighborhood to function properly.

By giving new team members a clear and accurate picture of your community's person-centered care approach and the various roles and responsibilities of team members in the Neighborhoods, you will equip them with the necessary tools to become fully integrated into the culture, which will significantly benefit and enhance the well-being of residents.

Defining the Culture of Your Community
REVIEW

- Describe the culture of your community and give examples of person-centered care practices.

- Familiarize new team members with the staff titles and nomenclature your community prefers.

- Educate new team members on daily routines and procedures.

- Define the role of each member of the Neighborhood or Household team.

- Create and foster a sense of teamwork.

- Explain how flexibility and cooperation are important qualities to help the team be successful.

- Stress the importance of building relationships in the Neighborhood with residents and co-workers.

- Provide an example of possible consequences of a lack of teamwork.

NOTES

_____

_____

_____

_____

_____

_____

_____

_____

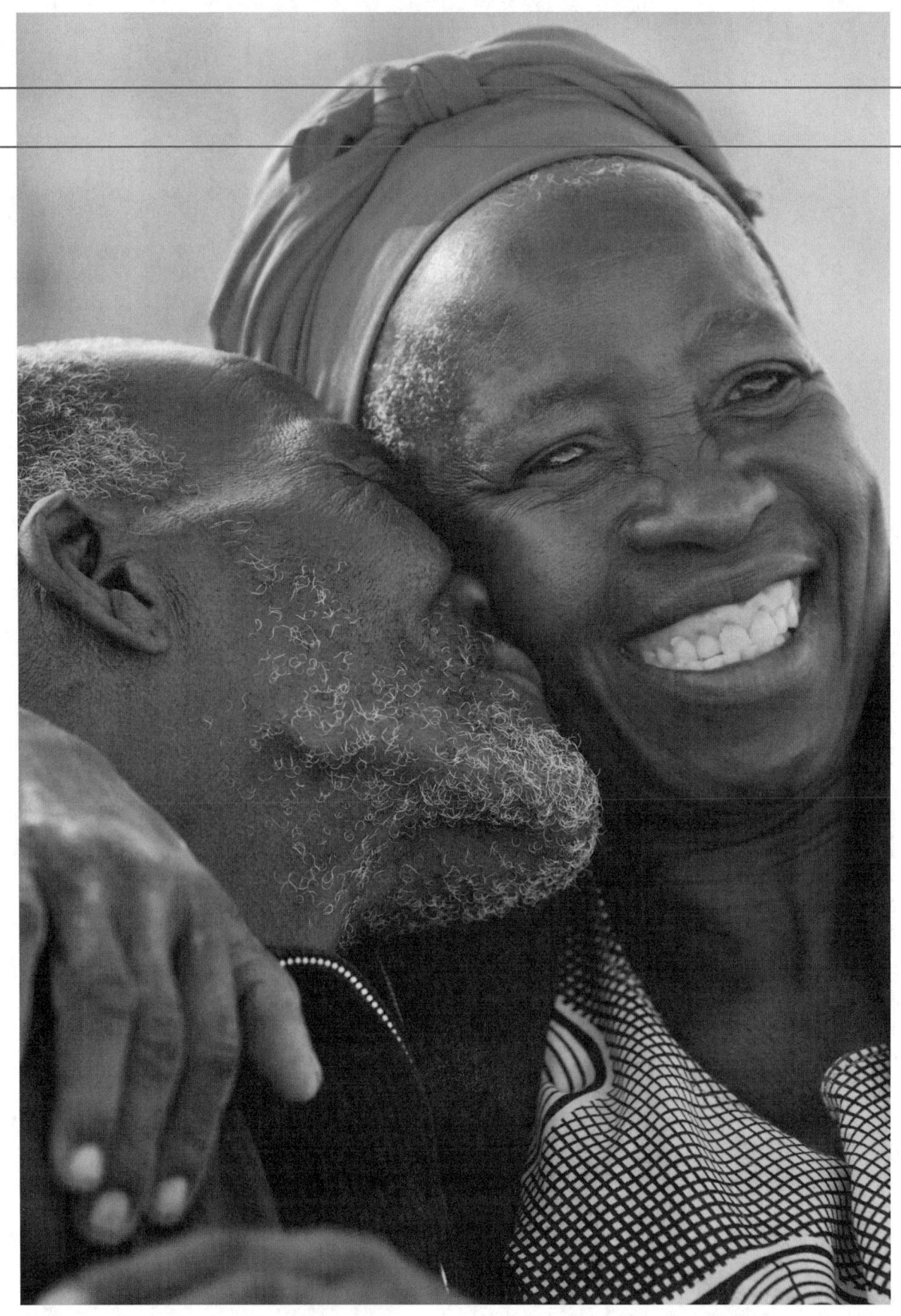

CHAPTER 5

Conducting the Orientation Program

As you prepare to conduct the orientation program, make sure everyone is aware in advance of the day, time, and location. To ensure that the program runs smoothly and efficiently, provide the attendees with information and materials in advance, such as paperwork they should bring with them, appropriate dress, available options for bringing or buying their lunch, and the approximate day and time the orientation will conclude. You may even want to suggest they bring a sweater or light jacket in case the room is too cool for their liking.

Prior to the orientees' arriving, arrange your classroom in a comfortable manner. If the class is small, have the group sit in a U-shape formation to promote eye contact and fellowship among attendees. For larger classes, consider using a "winged" arrangement to allow everyone the ability to see you and the presentations.

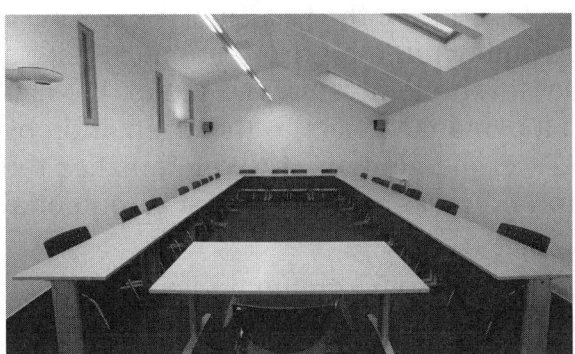 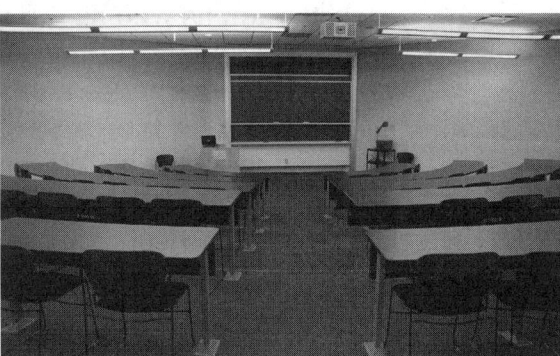

Prepare a name card to place in front of each orientee so that his or her name and title faces out toward the rest of the class. This will help the new team members to become familiar with each other. As mentioned in Chapter 2, print or label each orientee's name on the binder prepared for him or her and place it on the table or desk where he or she will sit. Assign seating to encourage interactions among different disciplines.

For example, instead of sitting nurses all together, intersperse them with CNAs or CMTs. This will create a sense of teamwork among the group, even if they will not be working on the same Neighborhood or shift.

Before starting the program, clearly express your position on the use of cell phones during class. Silenced phones sitting on a desk or tabletop are too much of a temptation to look at and pick up. Instead, ask each participant to silence his or her phone and put it away in a coat, purse, or backpack. Assure the group that you will allow for breaks to check messages and voicemails and that you prefer to have the class's undivided attention since the information presented is essential to their new jobs.

If refreshments will be provided, arrange them on a separate table that is attractively set with a covering as well as napkins, creamers, stirrers, and so forth. Providing coffee, hot or iced tea, and water is inexpensive and creates a welcoming, home-like atmosphere. Remember to announce at what times during the program breaks will be given, including when the group will break for lunch. And last but certainly not least, direct the class to where the restrooms are located.

As you prepare yourself for the orientation program, be very well versed in the material you will be presenting. Remember to avoid simply reading PowerPoint slides or speaking in a monotone voice. Interject personal experiences and invite the class to do the same so they are engaged and feel they are a part of the presentation.

When everyone is settled, give a brief outline of how the day will unfold. Review the agenda, including the title and approximate length of each session as well as the name and title of the presenter(s). It is best practice to involve other team members in the presentation to share a variety of experiences and maintain the interest of the group. In sharing their stories, the guests add a personal aspect to the orientation by speaking about their experiences in the community, which makes the presentations easier to relate to and more realistic. A list of potential guests and their speaking topics may include:

- *Director of nursing (DON):* In some communities, especially larger ones, staff rarely, if ever, see the DON. Night and evening shift staff have limited interaction with nursing management personnel, so it is important to meet and become acquainted with them during orientation. They should give a brief background on your community, touch lightly on overall person-centered care expectations, and welcome the new staff to share their concerns or comments at any time.

- *Nurse practitioners (NP) or physician's assistants (PA):* Depending on the nursing care team in your community, ask the

NP, PA, or even the Medical Director to introduce themselves to the new team members so they can put a name with a face and know who to contact should the need arise. Have them convey their preferred method of contact (e-mail, office phone, cell phone).

- *Dietitians:* It is important that new staff know who the dietitians are in your community so they feel comfortable approaching them with concerns about residents who present with difficulty swallowing or chewing. Have the dietitians explain the dietary options in a person-centered community and the residents' right to make choices about their meals. The dietitian can also address the importance of recording a new resident's weight at admission and periodically weighing residents according to your community's policy.

- *Social Services:* The Social Services department can address such topics as the move-in process, the importance of care plans, and the preservation of residents' rights. They can also talk about activities in the community and ways to engage with residents.

- *Therapy Services:* Therapists can present the transfer and lifting segment of the orientation. Their expertise and guidance will help new team members learn safe techniques and gain confidence when transferring residents. They can also explain the process for obtaining new referrals for physical therapy, speech therapy, and occupational therapy.

- *Activities:* Describe the types of person-centered activities that the community offers and invite the orientees to suggest new ideas for how to engage residents. If time permits, do a short, 10-minute activity with the new team members, such as a learning circle, in which a group of people comes together informally to discuss a specific topic. There is typically a facilitator for the learning circle. In this situation, the activities director can gather a group of orientees in a circle and choose a topic for them to share their thoughts on, such as favorite pets, vacations, hobbies, crafts, and so forth. It serves to create a common bond among the group members as well as to encourage engagement and communication.

- *Scheduler:* Discuss the on-time and paid time-off guidelines, overtime, scheduling details, and the process for calling off when staff are not able to come to work. Review the payday calendar so staff know when they can expect their paychecks.

- *Current staff:* Choose one person to invite from each of the different staff disciplines in your community to help present information included in the agenda. For example, when reviewing incontinence care, have a CNA come to the classroom and provide a demonstration using a mannequin. Ask a CMT to present the segment on proper use of a glucometer. An experienced nurse can show the orientees the proper way to document an assessment or perform an order entry.

- *Residents:* Invite a few residents to speak to the new team members. Have them talk about a typical day for them in Neighborhood and what they enjoy most about their lives in the community. Encourage them to ask questions of the orientees to learn about who will be taking care of them. Situate the residents in the center of the room and move the participants' chairs close around them to make it easier for them to engage in and hear the conversations. Resident guests have a huge impact on new team members and really drive home the message that they are the reason we have chosen to work in long-term care.

To begin the first day of orientation, start with introductions. Depending on the size of your group, there are various ways to break the ice. Keeping it informal eases the stress of making introductions and speaking about one's self. As the facilitator, begin by introducing yourself and offering a brief background of your training and what you do in the community. Also talk about for how long you have been employed by the organization, your chief role, and the reasons why you enjoy your job. Personal information should be kept to a minimum with the focus primarily on your association with the organization and the relationships you have built with co-workers and residents.

Next, have the new staff members introduce themselves. For small groups of four to five people, ask each person to state his or her name and title as well as share one personal fact with the group, such as place of birth, favorite flavor of ice cream, or if he or she has a pet. This is an easy way to create a sense of commonality among the participants.

For a larger group, time may not permit each person to talk about themselves. In this case, find creative ways to encourage sharing and camaraderie. One suggestion is a pairing exercise. Have two slips of paper, each with the same number on them for the amount of staff in the group. For example, if there are 10 people, have two slips with the number 1, two with the number 2, and so forth. If there are an uneven number of people in the class, include yourself as the facilitator in the exercise to round it out. Distribute the slips of paper to each member of the group. Instruct the class that during breaks and at lunch they are to seek out the person with their matching number and learn five things about him or her. During the final break of the day, the pair will stand up and share what they learned about the other person. This is a great exercise in relationship building. On the last day of orientation, encourage the group to remember this exercise and use it when they reach their Neighborhood or Household as a way to learn about the residents. Challenge them to learn at least five things about the residents each week. Doing so will help them to know the residents' likes and dislikes and find out things they may have in common with those in their care. Most of all, getting to know the residents will create an atmosphere of understanding and caring. Stress to the group that this is how person-centered care begins—by developing relationships and continuing to enhance them every day.

Proceed through the program with lecture, demonstrations, guests, and videos. Depending on the timing, it is a good idea to break up the classroom session with a walking tour of the community. This will give the class time to stretch their legs and see the environment they will be working in together. While touring the group, point out examples of a person-centered care approach they may not be readily aware of, such as:

- absence of overhead paging
- home-like atmosphere
- pleasant aroma of food being prepared in the Neighborhood
- absence of ringing call lights if pager system is used by staff
- well cared for appearance of residents
- informal interactions between care team members and residents

Stop along the way and introduce the new team members to current staff. Encourage staff to chat and give a brief description of their duties. Friendly and enthusiastic greetings from existing staff convey a hospitable and pleasant working atmosphere and help new staff feel welcomed. Observe whether orientees' appear comfortable and at ease interacting with residents during the tour through the Neighborhood. This may give insight into areas that may need to be addressed during the mentoring component of the orientation program.

Respect and honor an individual's learning ability and style in a person-centered manner. Employees will come from a wide variety of backgrounds and levels of experience. Newly graduated nurses may have difficulty grasping concepts. Competent, acute care nurses may face challenges adapting to a long-term care environment. At all levels of experience, learning a new computer system can be daunting. Be adaptable to the degrees of knowledge and aptitude among the orientees and teach to individual strengths and weaknesses accordingly. If a new team member requires a separate time for individualized training, make every attempt to accommodate his or her needs. While training, observe the class for those who are too timid or shy to voice their needs and approach them during a break. Offer your time in a quieter environment where they can feel relaxed and comfortable. Your concern will calm their stress and anxiety and help them transition into their new roles.

At the end of the first day, the CNAs will have completed their portion of the orientation program. Have them sign all of the necessary paperwork pertaining to them and then review what they submit for completeness. At this point, their mentors should arrive to introduce themselves and discuss where they will meet the next day at the start of the shift. This is also the time to give the new CNAs a copy of their schedules so they know in advance when they will be working. Before they leave, wish them well and encourage them to contact you at any time if they have questions or concerns. And be sure to give each new CNA your contact information, including phone number and email address.

Inform the remaining orientees in the class of the time to meet again in the morning. Encourage them to arrive well rested and ready to learn more about their new roles. Offer praise for their attentiveness and be enthusiastic about the remaining topics. Lastly, make sure all of the trash is cleaned up and the table and chairs are reset for the next day.

On the second day of orientation, continue working through the agenda with the remaining orientees. As the class thins out, you may choose to rearrange the seating to accommodate a smaller group. When each discipline completes their portion, repeat the same process of signing paperwork, meeting mentors, and sending them on their way. With the initial orientation program complete, the new staff will have a solid foundation on which to build their new careers in your community. Chapter 6 discusses the next step in the orientation process: the "hands-on" training with mentors.

Conducting the Orientation Program
REVIEW

- Review the agenda with the orientees, including when and where to meet for each session.

- Arrange the classroom according to the size of the group.

- Print or label each orientee's name on the binder prepared for him or her and place it on the table or desk where he or she will sit.

- Provide refreshments and announce when breaks can be taken.

- Invite guest staff to present portions of the program.

- Ask each orientee to introduce him- or herself to the group and encourage sharing and camaraderie.

- Take the new hires on a walking tour of the community, including meeting current staff along the way.

- As each discipline completes their portion of the orientation, have them sign their paperwork and meet their mentors.

- Recognize and respect varied learning styles and teach accordingly.

NOTES

_____

_____

_____

_____

_____

_____

_____

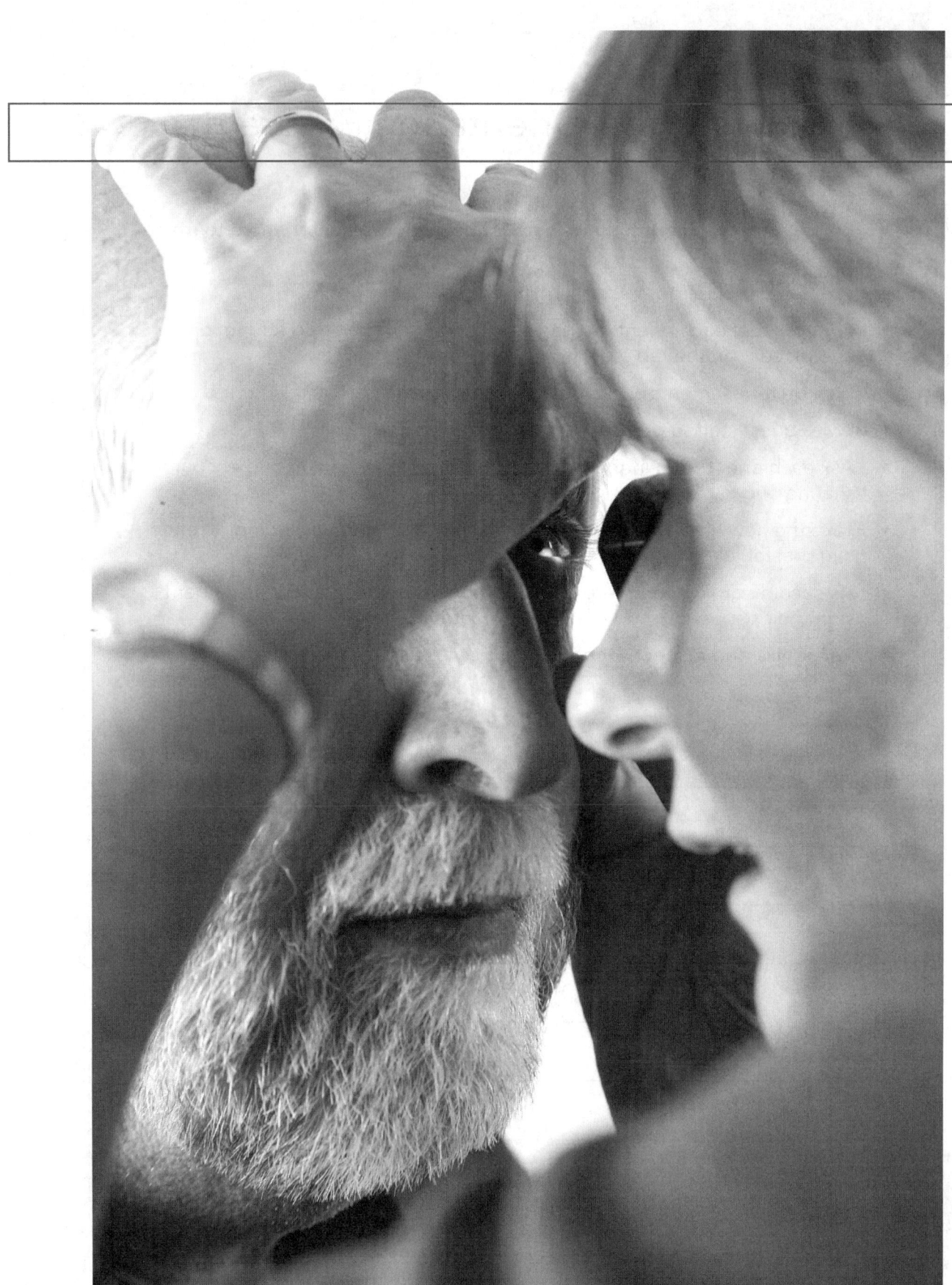

CHAPTER 6

Skills Testing for New and Existing Staff

Before the new hires are allowed to begin working independently in your community, their skills must first be tested. Even the most experienced nurse or nurse's aide will need to be tested for several reasons, such as the following:

- They may not have used certain skill sets for a long time.
- They may have never performed certain tasks or employed certain skills.
- The policies and procedures for your community may differ from other healthcare settings.
- Inaccurate or unsafe methods of performing tasks will need to be identified and corrected.

There are two ways to test the skills of new hires as part of the orientation program. One method of skills testing is to have a lab set up in a classroom with a life-size, anatomically correct mannequin. The other is to have the mentors verify the orientees' skills when working together with them.

For the classroom setting, have all of the necessary supplies at hand for each skills test. Give each orientee a packet with the skills checklist that pertains to their discipline. If time allows and the group size is not too large, demonstrate each skill and then have each orientee perform a return demonstration. For larger classes, you can have orientees team up and work together in performing the return demonstrations.

The skills that need to be tested include, but are not limited to, the following:

- hand-washing
- infection control
- transfer and lifting techniques

- pericare
- oral hygiene care
- applying TED hose
- using personal protective equipment
- catheter care
- post-mortem care

Each skill should have a demonstration check-off list for the instructor to use in testing whether proper procedure was followed. Create each checklist using your community's policy and procedure manual or your state's CNA handbook. Include as many of the basic skills as you feel are necessary, depending on the class, resources, and time limitations. See the Skills Demonstration Checklist at the end of the chapter, which is an example of a checklist for hand-washing. You can use this style of form as a template for testing other skills. The instructor will observe the orientee, mark the check-off list, and sign the form if the skill was performed correctly and according to your community's policy and procedure. The orientee will also sign the form.

For the hand-washing skill, you should have a black light kit available to ensure hands are thoroughly washed and clean. The kit contains a gel substance that is applied to the hands and that glows under the black light. After the orientee washes his or her hands, shine the light on both hands to make sure all of the gel has been removed. Usually the areas surrounding the fingernails and underneath rings are not sufficiently cleaned.

To begin skills testing, review with the orientees the checklist for the first skill to be tested and the proper steps to be performed, and then ask each orientee to complete the skill. After all of the skills are tested during orientation, the mentors will then observe how the new team members perform each skill in the Neighborhoods to ensure they continue to practice proper techniques.

For nurses and CMTs, additional skills testing is needed for the areas of practice for which they will be responsible. Some of these skills include the following:

- nebulizer and inhaler treatment administration
- total parenteral nutrition
- glucose monitoring
- insulin administration
- administering various forms of medications, including intravenous, transdermal, subcutaneous, intramuscular, sublingual, topical, and ophthalmic and otic drops

- tracheostomy care
- nasogastric tube care
- ventilator care and monitoring

Create the skills list based on the services offered by your community and the guidelines for each individual discipline's scope of practice. See, for example, the sample Medication Administration Test at the end of the chapter, which can be used to test an orientee's knowledge of administering medications. Also at the end of the chapter is a more general Skills Demonstration Checklist for testing new hires that has a section for CNAs and CMTs as well as one for RNs and LPNs. A sample Resident Transfer Training Checklist and Gait Belt Compliance Form can also be found at the end of the chapter for testing new team members during the orientation process.

In addition to testing the skills of new team members, every community should offer ongoing skills training for all staff. It is essential to keep everyone's skills in line with the most current changes to local, state, and federal regulations so that existing staff can in turn properly train new team members. This also ensures that everyone is following the same methods of practice uniformly throughout the community. Monthly in-services and annual skills fairs are excellent ways to offer skills practice opportunities to your staff. Monthly staff meetings should include a review of a skill that is repeatedly performed incorrectly or a skill that the staff requests more training on.

Annual skills fair days are a great way to cover many topics in just one day. Set up several stations in an auditorium or large conference room and give short presentations on skills you have identified that staff need more education on. The previous year's annual state survey will provide insight into areas of concern that should be addressed. Make the skills fair day fun and exciting for staff. Choose a theme, such as a Hawaiian luau, sports, or characters from a movie. Enlist the help of leadership within the community and volunteers to make the day successful. Provide refreshments and small prizes for each team member who successfully completes his or her assigned skills test.

The following are some tips for a baseball-themed skills fair day for nursing:

- Title your skills fair day "Take Me Out to the Ballgame."
- Decorate the room to resemble a baseball diamond.
- If you have a local team, decorate the room with its logo or colors.
- Have a different topic at each "base."

- Give the attendees a "scorecard" showing which bases they must visit.
- Place instructors at each base to present a 10–15 minute presentation on their assigned topic.
- The instructors will give the attendees a short test (5–7 questions) at the end of each presentation.
- The instructors will sign off on each attendee's scorecard when he or she has successfully completed a test. The scorecards can be placed in the employee's file as verification of skills competency (see the sample scorecard and program at the end of the chapter).
- Have popcorn, peanuts, and soft drinks for refreshments.
- Encourage staff to attend dressed in casual clothes with a baseball jersey or shirt.
- All instructors should be dressed in baseball attire.
- Solicit various departments in the community to donate prizes, such as themed baskets or baseball tickets, if there is a local team. Prizes can also include free lunches in the cafeteria.

Be sure to take pictures of staff actively participating in the activities. If you have a newsletter or website, post the pictures along with the names of staff who won any attendance prizes or giveaways. Annual skills fair days satisfy regulatory requirements, engage leadership with staff, and reinforce necessary skills. They are also just one more way to provide a person-centered learning opportunity for your team.

The orientees are now ready to start working in the community. The next chapter describes the process for introducing new hires to the Neighborhood and the important role mentors playing in helping them get acclimated.

Skills Testing for New and Existing Staff
REVIEW

- Skills testing is necessary to ensure all new team members are capable and knowledgeable.

- Test skills related to each discipline.

- Skills testing can be done by setting up a lab with a life-size, anatomically correct mannequin, or by having the mentors verify the orientees' skills when working together with them.

- Document each orientee's return demonstration using a skills demonstration checklist related to each discipline and keep a copy in his or her employee file.

- Continuing education and skills fairs help keep skills current and accurate.

- Create a fun theme and atmosphere for annual skills fairs and acknowledge participants in your community newsletter or website.

NOTES

_____

_____

_____

_____

_____

_____

_____

_____

Skills Demonstration Checklist

NAME _____

TITLE _____

SKILL PERFORMED _Hand-washing_ CATEGORY _Infection control_

PROCEDURE	P	NR
1. Water at sink at recommended temperature (hot without harm to skin)	☐	☐
2. Hands and wrists thoroughly wet	☐	☐
3. Soap applied to hands	☐	☐
4. All surfaces of hand lathered well, including wrists and fingers	☐	☐
5. Friction applied to all surfaces for at least 20 seconds	☐	☐
6. Fingernails on each hand cleaned by rubbing vigorously against opposite palm	☐	☐
7. Hands and wrists rinsed in a downward motion while maintaining hands lower than elbows	☐	☐
8. Clean paper towel used to thoroughly dry hands and wrists	☐	☐
9. Clean paper towel used to turn off faucet	☐	☐
10. No surface touched after hands cleaned	☐	☐
11. If necessary, clean paper towel used to open door	☐	☐

P = Passed   NR = Needs Review

_____   _____
Employee's Signature   Date

_____   _____
Instructor's Signature   Date

Medication Administration Test

NAME _____

DATE _____

1. List the six rights of medication administration:

   a. _____ d. _____

   b. _____ e. _____

   c. _____ f. _____

2. A resident's order reads: 60 mgs Diovan, p.o., daily. Only 40 mg tablets are available. How would you administer this medication?

3. A resident has an order for 500 mls of IV infusion to run over a period of 12 hours. What is the hourly rate of infusion?

4. What are the common side effects of Digoxin? What vital signs should be monitored?

5. How many kilograms is a resident weighing 240 pounds?

6. Who should reconcile controlled substances and how often?

7. What is the recommended wait time between administering two different types of eye drops?

8. What is the procedure for a resident who refuses medication?

Skills Demonstration Checklist (CNA/CMT)

NAME _____

TITLE _____ NEIGHBORHOOD _____

To be completed by mentor. Please submit completed forms to Nursing Supervisor.

CLINICAL SKILLS		MEETS EXPECTATIONS	NEEDS IMPROVEMENT	DATE
Hand-washing		☐	☐	
Infection control		☐	☐	
Personal protective equipment:	Donning	☐	☐	
	Removing	☐	☐	
Pericare female		☐	☐	
Pericare male		☐	☐	
Catheter care:	Foley bag	☐	☐	
	Leg bag	☐	☐	
Correct use of diet cards		☐	☐	
Follows fall protocol and procedure		☐	☐	
Obtains and documents vital signs properly		☐	☐	
Obtains and documents weights properly		☐	☐	
Obtains and documents heights properly		☐	☐	
Ostomy care		☐	☐	
Baths, showers, whirlpool		☐	☐	
Skin care		☐	☐	
Resident transfers		☐	☐	
Proper use of gait belt		☐	☐	
Lifts:	Stander	☐	☐	
	Full mechanical	☐	☐	

INSULIN ADMINISTRATION (CMT ONLY)	MEETS EXPECTATIONS	NEEDS IMPROVEMENT	DATE
Blood glucose monitoring	☐	☐	
Glucometer quality control procedures	☐	☐	
Medication preparation	☐	☐	
Medication administration	☐	☐	
Medication documentation	☐	☐	
Correct identification of resident	☐	☐	
Medication destruction	☐	☐	
Medication order/refill	☐	☐	

continued

Skills Demonstration Checklist (CNA/CMT) *cont.*

COMMUNICATION/DOCUMENTATION SKILLS	MEETS EXPECTATIONS	NEEDS IMPROVEMENT	DATE
Communicates important information to nurse and/or supervisors	☐	☐	
Addresses residents appropriately	☐	☐	
Shows respect for residents and honors their dignity	☐	☐	
Documents resident data accurately	☐	☐	
Performs walking rounds at the start and end of each shift	☐	☐	
Manages time efficiently to complete all duties and documentation in a timely manner	☐	☐	
Seeks assistance when needed to perform skills efficiently and correctly	☐	☐	
Proficient with EMR documentation	☐	☐	

NEIGHBORHOOD ORIENTATION	MEETS EXPECTATIONS	NEEDS IMPROVEMENT	DATE
Understands emergency codes	☐	☐	
Fire safety (equipment location and use)	☐	☐	
Utility rooms (clean and dirty)	☐	☐	
Biohazard trash/room	☐	☐	
Oxygen supply room	☐	☐	
Emergency procedures/ambu-bag location	☐	☐	
Call light system	☐	☐	
Nourishment area/kitchen	☐	☐	
Uses proper telephone etiquette	☐	☐	
Laundry room	☐	☐	
Resident charges	☐	☐	
Time clocks	☐	☐	
Lunch room	☐	☐	
Neighborhood staff schedule	☐	☐	

_____   _____
Mentor's Signature   Date

_____   _____
Orientee's Signature   Date

_____   _____
Supervisor's Signature   Date

Skills Demonstration Checklist (RN/LPN)

NAME _____

TITLE _____ NEIGHBORHOOD _____

To be completed by mentor. Please submit completed forms to Nursing Supervisor.

CLINICAL SKILLS		MEETS EXPECTATIONS	NEEDS IMPROVEMENT	DATE
Hand-washing		☐	☐	
Infection control		☐	☐	
Personal protective equipment:	Donning	☐	☐	
	Removing	☐	☐	
Pericare female		☐	☐	
Pericare male		☐	☐	
Catheter care:	Foley bag	☐	☐	
	Leg bag	☐	☐	
Correct use of diet cards		☐	☐	
Follows fall protocol and procedure		☐	☐	
Obtains and documents vital signs properly		☐	☐	
Obtains and documents heights and weights properly		☐	☐	
Ostomy care		☐	☐	
Baths, showers, whirlpool		☐	☐	
Resident transfers		☐	☐	
Proper use of gait belt		☐	☐	
Lifts:	Stander	☐	☐	
	Full mechanical	☐	☐	

PHARMACY	MEETS EXPECTATIONS	NEEDS IMPROVEMENT	DATE
Verify orders and maintain medication list	☐	☐	
Refill medications	☐	☐	
Monitor drug expiration dates	☐	☐	
Prepare and administer oral medications	☐	☐	
Perform injections properly	☐	☐	
Apply transdermal medications properly	☐	☐	

continued

Skills Demonstration Checklist (RN/LPN) *cont.*

LABORATORY/RADIOLOGY	MEETS EXPECTATIONS	NEEDS IMPROVEMENT	DATE
Collect urine/stool specimen	☐	☐	
Enter orders, document results, notify physician and other responsible parties in a timely manner	☐	☐	

ENTERAL FEEDING	MEETS EXPECTATIONS	NEEDS IMPROVEMENT	DATE
Enter orders accurately	☐	☐	
Perform feeding according to protocol	☐	☐	
Document accurately	☐	☐	

INSULIN ADMINISTRATION	MEETS EXPECTATIONS	NEEDS IMPROVEMENT	DATE
Blood glucose monitoring	☐	☐	
Glucometer quality control procedures	☐	☐	
Medication preparation	☐	☐	
Medication administration	☐	☐	
Medication documentation	☐	☐	
Correct identification of resident	☐	☐	
Medication destruction	☐	☐	
Medication order/refill	☐	☐	

SKIN AND WOUND CARE	MEETS EXPECTATIONS	NEEDS IMPROVEMENT	DATE
Enter orders accurately	☐	☐	
Perform treatments properly	☐	☐	
Document accurately	☐	☐	

COMMUNICATION/DOCUMENTATION SKILLS	MEETS EXPECTATIONS	NEEDS IMPROVEMENT	DATE
Communicates important information to physicians, NPs, supervisors	☐	☐	
Addresses residents appropriately	☐	☐	
Shows respect for residents and honors their dignity	☐	☐	
Performs walking rounds at the start and end of each shift	☐	☐	
Manages time efficiently to complete all duties and documentation in a timely manner	☐	☐	

continued

Skills Demonstration Checklist (RN/LPN) *cont.*

COMMUNICATION/DOCUMENTATION SKILLS	MEETS EXPECTATIONS	NEEDS IMPROVEMENT	DATE
Seeks assistance when needed to perform skills efficiently and correctly	☐	☐	
Delegates work to appropriate staff	☐	☐	
Supervises CNAs and CMTs	☐	☐	
Promotes teamwork on Neighborhood	☐	☐	
Ensures call lights are answered in a timely manner	☐	☐	
Communicates well with family members	☐	☐	
Proficient with EMR documentation	☐	☐	

NEIGHBORHOOD ORIENTATION	MEETS EXPECTATIONS	NEEDS IMPROVEMENT	DATE
Understands emergency codes	☐	☐	
Fire safety (equipment location and use)	☐	☐	
Utility rooms (clean and dirty)	☐	☐	
Biohazard trash/room	☐	☐	
Oxygen supply room	☐	☐	
Emergency procedures/ambu-bag location	☐	☐	
Call light system	☐	☐	
Nourishment area/kitchen	☐	☐	
Uses proper telephone etiquette	☐	☐	
Laundry room	☐	☐	
Resident charges	☐	☐	
Time clocks	☐	☐	
Lunch room	☐	☐	
Neighborhood staff schedule	☐	☐	

_____   _____
Mentor's Signature   Date

_____   _____
Orientee's Signature   Date

_____   _____
Supervisor's Signature   Date

Resident Transfer Training Checklist

NAME _____

DEPARTMENT _____

TITLE _____

DATE OF HIRE _____

Instructions for the following were reviewed during orientation:

1. Proper posture when transferring a resident

2. Using a gait belt properly

3. Walking a resident:
   a. with a cane
   b. with a walker

4. Transferring a resident:
   a. from bed to wheelchair
   b. from bed to standing
   c. from wheelchair to commode or toilet

5. Assisting a resident who is prone to falling

6. How to properly position a resident:
   a. in bed
   b. in a chair

I confirm that I have been taught the techniques listed above and have full understanding of the proper procedures.

_____   _____
Orientee's Signature   Date

I certify that the above-named employee has successfully demonstrated proper technique, as evidenced by return demonstration.

_____   _____
Instructor's Signature   Date

Gait Belt Compliance Form

NAME _____

DEPARTMENT _____

TITLE _____

DATE OF HIRE _____

I have been trained on the proper use of a gait belt and understand the necessary safety measures to employ when transferring a resident.

I understand that a gait belt is considered part of my uniform to be worn at all times while providing resident care.

I understand that failure to wear a gait belt and use it when it is appropriate to do so will result in my being subject to appropriate disciplinary action, up to and including termination.

_____   _____
Orientee's Signature   Date

_____   _____
Instructor's Signature   Date

"Take Me Out to the Ballgame"
Annual Skills Fair Day

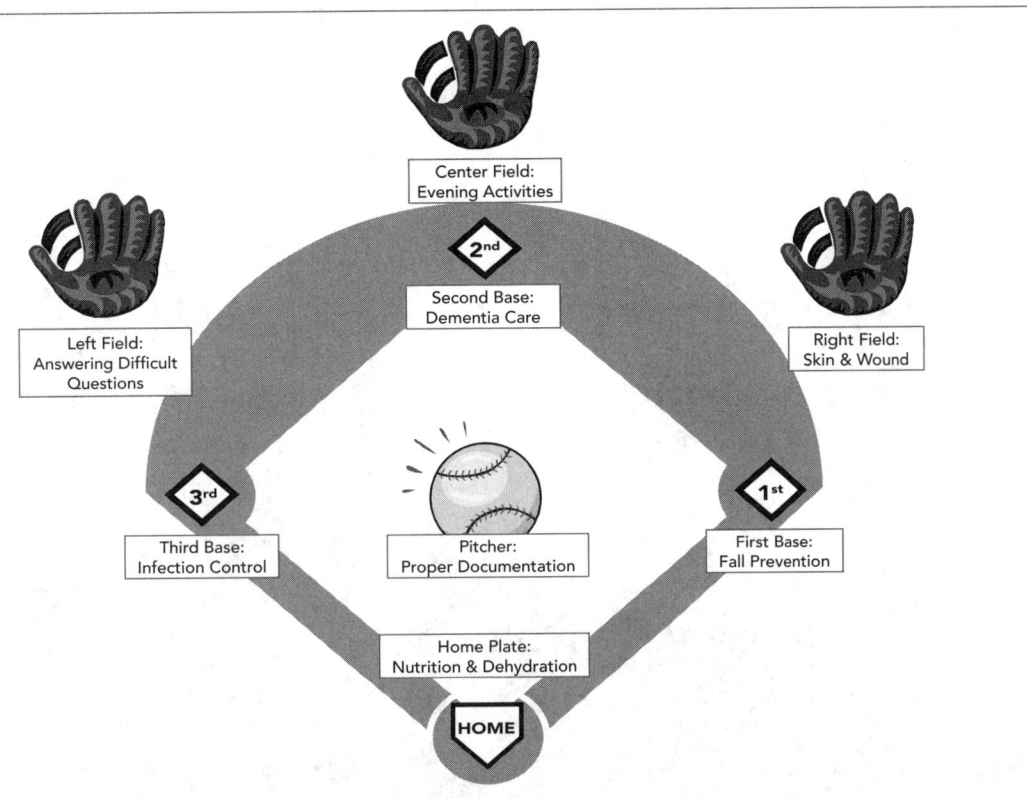

PLAYER NAME

_____

POSITION (TITLE)

_____

☐   HOME RUN!

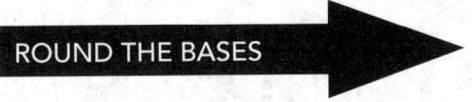

Take a turn pitching and in the outfield.

Visit each table in your line-up and complete the post-test. Don't forget to visit the refreshment stand!!

TOPIC	WHO ATTENDS	COMPLETED
First Base: Fall Prevention	Nurses, CNAs, CMTs	☐
Second Base: Dementia Care	Nurses, CNAs, CMTs, Homemakers	☐
Third Base: Infection Control	Nurses, CNAs, CMTs, Homemakers	☐
Pitcher: Proper Documentation	Nurses	☐
Right Field: Skin & Wound	Nurses, CNAs, CMTs	☐
Center Field: Evening Activities	Nurses, CNAs, CMTs, Homemakers	☐
Left Field: Answering Difficult Questions	Nurses, CNAs, CMTs, Homemakers	☐
Home Plate: Nutrition & Dehydration	Nurses, CNAs, CMTs, Homemakers	☐

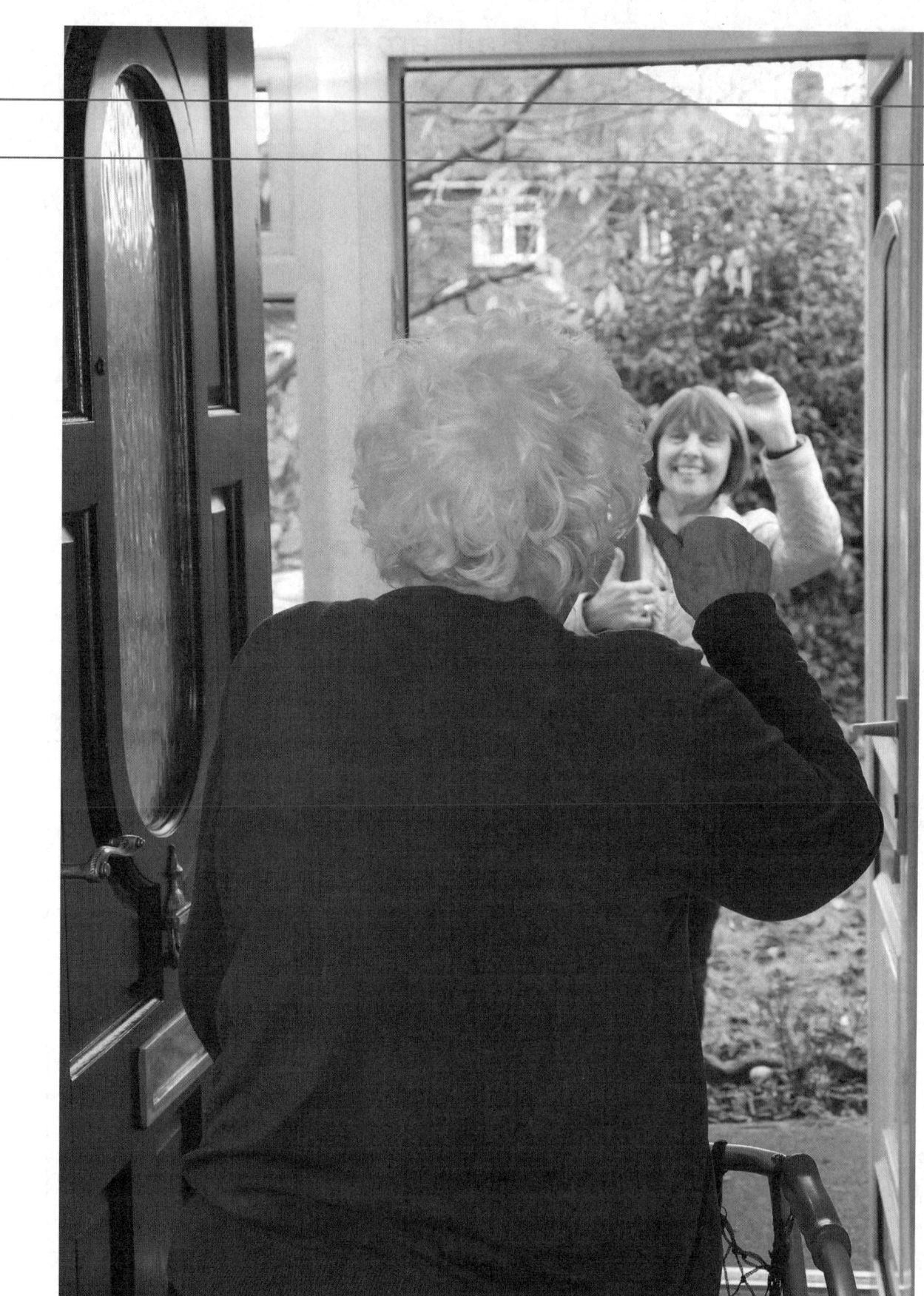

CHAPTER 7

The First Days on the Neighborhood

More often than not, a new employee is plunged unceremoniously into the first day of work without the benefit of someone to formally greet or show him or her around the Neighborhood and community. The anxiety and uncertainty of starting a new job is exacerbated by the sense of awkwardness and loneliness often experienced by being the new kid on the block. For the orientee, adapting to a new community is filled with stressors of different types, including the following:

- knowing where to park
- knowing where to report and how to clock in
- where to eat meals
- remembering the names of new co-workers
- learning job duties and policies and procedures
- learning a new computer documentation system
- knowing the various vendors and service providers
- meeting and becoming acquainted with the residents for whom they will be providing care and their families
- understanding the culture of the community

In a person-centered care environment, the first impression conveyed to the new team member should be warm, friendly, and inviting. Mentors play an important role in this regard in the first days on the Neighborhood for new hires. Since our expectation is to create a sense of family in each Neighborhood or Household, mentors should greet their new co-workers in the same manner they would welcome a guest in their home. Mentors need to send the message through their words and actions that they are truly excited the new hires have chosen to become a part of the team.

As part of an orientee's first day, the mentor should plan to facilitate a learning circle that will include all of the team members in the Neighborhood. Have each person introduce him- or herself and briefly share what his or her background and history is within the community. Allow the new team members to share as much or as little as they choose. Having the existing nursing team members take just 10 or 15 minutes out of their day to engage in a friendly atmosphere promotes acceptance and shows the orientees that their new co-workers genuinely care about their well-being. During the learning circle, also take a moment to restate the organization's mission statement and reinforce how each team member plays an integral part in upholding the community's values and beliefs.

Mentors help orientees become acclimated to their new surroundings and ease the anxiety of the first day. They also play an important role in fostering successful relationships between existing and new team members. It is essential to organize and coordinate designated mentors who will meet and greet all new orientees prior to their first day in the Neighborhood. Lack of preplanning sets up both the mentor and mentee for failure. Planning ahead avoids the unfortunate scenario played out all too often whereby an experienced staff member is chosen at random to serve as a mentor. Upon arriving for his or her shift, the staff member is told he or she will guide a new hire for the day. Without the courtesy of any advance notice, he or she is perturbed at the thought of training a new co-worker. The imposition is not well received and the staff member's sense of frustration is not conducive to extending a warm welcome to the new team member. The new co-worker in turn feels he or she is an imposition and an unwelcomed challenge. The two begin their shift under awkward and strained circumstances, and the first impression is one of disorganized chaos, which leads the new co-worker to wonder what lies ahead.

The person-centered approach to welcoming new staff takes into consideration both the experienced staff member and the new team member. It is preplanned and structured so there are no surprises for either person. When choosing a mentor, try to determine if he or she would be compatible with a new hire. To achieve a successful mentor–mentee relationship, follow these steps:

1. The Human Resources representative and staff development coordinator/educator meet prior to the first day of orientation to determine a training schedule.

2. An appropriate mentor for each new team member is chosen based on the prospective mentor's level of experience and availability.

3. The orientee and mentor are introduced to each other prior to the first day of work to allow time to get acquainted. The orientee can anticipate a familiar face as opposed to just showing up to work and knowing no one.

4. The mentor and orientee determine where and when they will meet at the beginning of the shift.

5. The mentor facilitates a learning circle with the other team members in the Neighborhood.

6. The mentor guides the orientee through the first day, introducing him or her to staff, residents, supervisors, and so forth.

7. The mentor and orientee continue on together through each day of training until the orientee is comfortable and capable enough to work independently.

This guideline helps the orientee become familiar with the Household and staff and eliminates the feeling of being alone to fend for oneself, which can lead to mistakes and poor outcomes.

As the first few days proceed, the mentor will give the orientee an overview of his or her new role and duties. The mentor will also show the orientee the Neighborhood where he or she will work and surrounding places, such as the medication and supply rooms, kitchen and dining rooms, laundry and clean/dirty utility rooms, lunch and break rooms, and location of lockers or coat closets. The mentor will extend the tour beyond the orientee's work area to the remainder of the Neighborhood, such as the location of the Human Resources department, business offices, and the immediate supervisor's office.

As the orientee's level of comfort increases, the mentor will begin to delve into the more detailed aspects of the job, allow the new team member to perform the daily tasks related to his or her position, and observe and provide guidance. While working together throughout the day, the mentor should note the orientee's skills level and complete any appropriate skills competency checklists. Areas that need improvement or further training should be addressed immediately to avoid having an orientee develop bad habits or perform procedural techniques improperly. It is also important to encourage new team members to absorb as much as they can during the orientation period when they have the benefit of one-on-one training with a mentor. Reassure them that this is the time to ask questions and test their skills. By expending as much attention and effort as they can during this period, the orientees will learn the necessary skills to be successful.

With the anxiety of being new and unaccustomed to their environment alleviated, the orientees are now able to absorb new concepts and procedures in a relaxed manner. Their rate of success is greatly enhanced and they are off to a good start. Chapter 8 discusses the next step in the orientation process, which is to help the new team members to form and nurture strong relationships with the residents they will be caring for.

The First Days on the Neighborhood
REVIEW

- Create a welcoming atmosphere for new team members to help ease their stress and anxiety during the orientation process as they become familiar with new staff and their surroundings.

- Facilitate a learning circle that includes all current team members in the welcoming process and to show you all care.

- Preplan the designation of a mentor prior to an orientee's first day.

- Encourage new team members to absorb as much as they can during the orientation period when they have the benefit of one-on-one training with a mentor so they learn the necessary skills to be successful.

NOTES

_____

_____

_____

_____

_____

_____

_____

_____

_____

_____

_____

_____

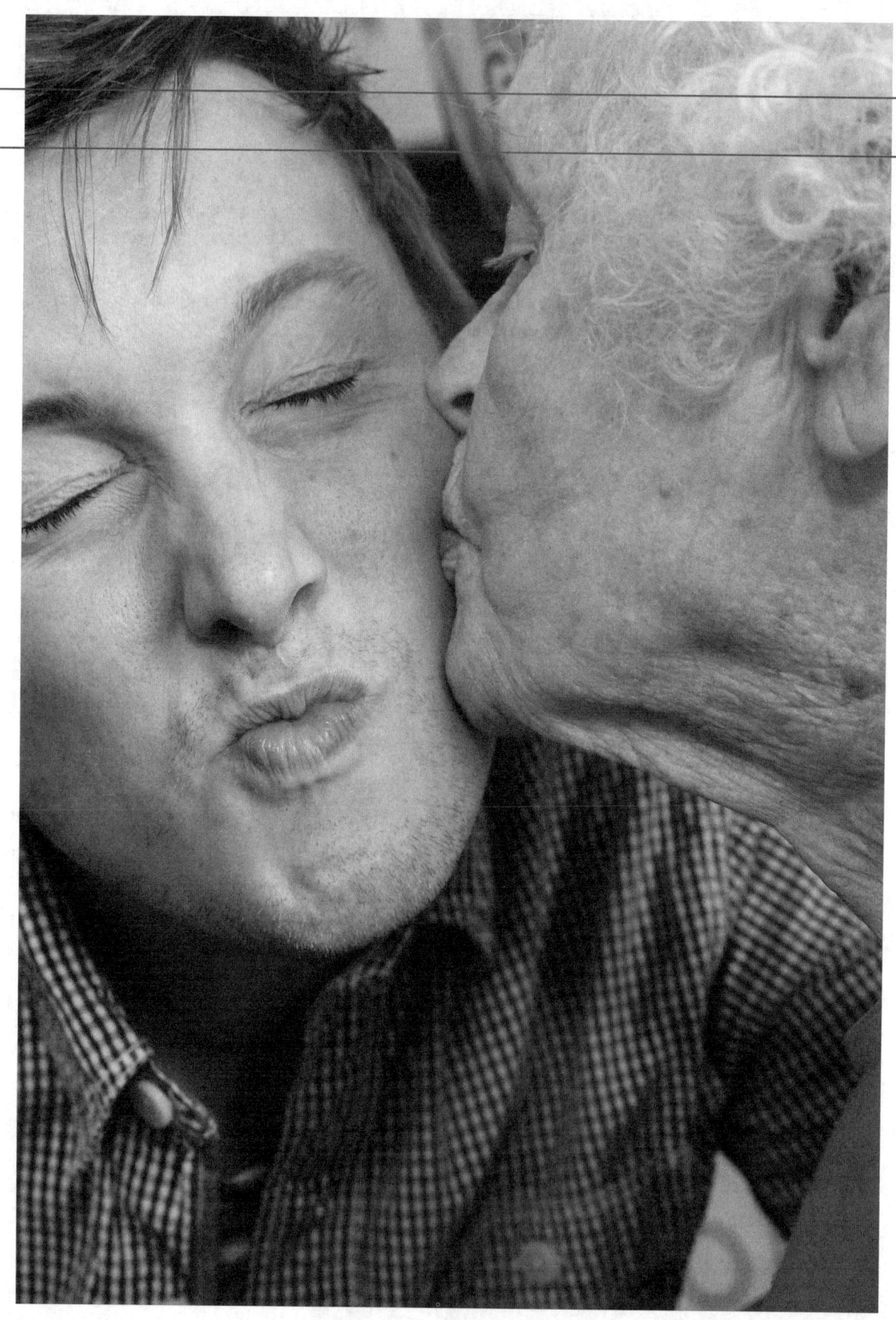

CHAPTER 8

Building Successful Relationships

At the heart of person-centered care is forming and nurturing strong relationships with those being cared for. It is absolutely essential to learn as much as possible about each individual in order to provide care that is consistent with his or her wishes and desires. For example, knowing a resident's meal preferences, such as disliking scrambled eggs for breakfast, will avoid many problems, including the resident refusing a meal, unexpected weight loss, and difficult confrontations between the resident and staff. In contrast, when the resident's food choices are recorded and posted, the dietary team knows exactly what to serve, which in turn creates a satisfactory mealtime experience.

Acknowledging patterns, personal habits, and traditions is equally as important. A retired nurse who spent her entire career working the night shift is not apt to go to bed at 7:00 p.m. with the rest of the residents in the Neighborhood. Rather than attempt to change her lifelong routine either by insisting she go to bed early or attempting to give her a sedative, the staff should honor her choice of when she wants to go to bed. Prepare an area where she can relax before going to bed, perhaps to watch television or read a book without disturbing other residents who are sleeping. If staff have some idle time, they can ask her if she would like some company and, if so, they can visit with her and provide companionship. During the daytime when she would rather be sleeping, try to maintain a quiet and dark room where she can rest peacefully.

Teach your staff that honoring a person's wishes encompasses many factors, such as upbringing, religious beliefs, dietary habits, and personal preferences. Residents who lived during the Great Depression have very different views and attitudes than the younger generation who are now caring for them. During a time when commodities such as food and clean water were at a premium, these residents developed habits such as eating modestly and bathing only once a week. If your community has guidelines that state the resident must bathe twice weekly, there is bound to be conflict. Instead, create a person-centered care plan that states the resident may have a sponge bath during the week and a full tub bath on Saturdays. In this instance, everyone wins; the resident can continue to do as she has done in the past without being made to feel as though she is doing something wrong, and the staff are able to complete their tasks in an amiable and productive fashion. Encourage staff to allow residents to make choices that will make them happy.

Modesty is often a concern for older residents. It is very uncomfortable to not only undress in front of others, but to be bathed by someone else, especially a new caregiver. Some residents may prefer not to be cared for by a staff member of the opposite sex. Communicate to staff that they should strive to understand the feelings of each resident in their care and uphold his or her morals and values. If a male care companion is available, pair him with a gentleman resident who is embarrassed to have a female aide attend to his personal needs. Update the resident's care plan so that everyone involved in his care is aware of his choices.

At a time in their lives when residents have reduced a lifetime of collecting personal belongings into a single, small room, possibly shared with a stranger, it is very difficult to reconcile losing control over one's living space. Learning the answers to personal lifestyle questions will help staff learn the preferences of those in their care and thereby enhance the living experience of residents. Residents not only feel more at home, but the caregiver bond is also strengthened. The following are a few suggestions for how to create an atmosphere that evokes positive feelings for residents:

- Incorporate personal items of sentimental significance into the décor of the resident's room to create a connection with his or her past.
- Place photographs and mementos in an area where they can be easily seen when the resident is in his or her room.
- Hang a bulletin board to display art or schoolwork from a resident's loved ones.
- Create a shadow box filled with keepsakes that are of sentimental value to the resident. Place it either inside his or her room or just outside the door. This will also help the resident differentiate his or her room from other rooms that may look identical.
- Play a resident's favorite music or involve the person in a game or activity to help lift his or her spirits if he or she is feeling sad, lonely, or depressed.

To help build new relationships, an in-depth interview at the time of admission will answer many questions and become the key to unlocking the mysteries that make each resident unique. It will also equip staff with the tools they need to provide care in a person-centered manner. In the admission packet for each new resident should be a copy of *The*

Story of Me, which includes a list of some of the questions that should be asked when a new resident comes to live in your community (a sample form can be found at the end the chapter). It should be kept in the resident's chart or file where it can be readily reviewed by staff. If necessary, have a family member assist in completing the form. *The Story of Me* focuses on the resident's choices and creative ways to honor them.

As staff become familiar with residents and learn about their pasts, they, too, can share information about themselves. Residents will feel they truly are a part of a family when they know about their caregivers. Set guidelines as to what information is appropriate to share and what is unacceptable, such as the following:

- Staff are encouraged to share:
    - family information (number of children, grandchildren, siblings)
    - hobbies and sports
    - schooling and studies
    - family and holiday traditions
    - personal goals and accomplishments

- Staff should refrain from discussing:
    - personal financial or marital problems
    - negative personal information (car problems, family members in trouble)
    - disturbing information or upsetting current events
    - disgruntled attitudes toward co-workers or the community
    - technology that is foreign or incomprehensible to the resident

When staff share pleasant, upbeat details about their lives, residents feel connected with their caregivers and a strong bond is created. When a mutual fondness and interest exists between staff and residents, the process of providing care proceeds at a more relaxed and comfortable pace. In knowing more about their caregivers, residents trust them and have confidence in their abilities. Staff members are apt to provide the best care possible to residents and take pride and comfort in knowing they can help to brighten their day while attending to their needs.

Family members benefit from staff-to-resident relationships as well. They have a greater sense of trust when they know the staff who are taking care of their loved one are genuinely interested in them. Often there is a sense of guilt or remorse when placing loved ones in a long-term care facility, or care center. Family members also experience feelings of inadequacy in not being able to provide care at home or of letting down a parent who has raised and taken care of them. These feelings are eased when they realize that staff will care for their loved one in a loving, considerate, and respectful manner. Knowing their family member is treated with compassion, affection, and understanding eases the stress and burden of regret.

Ask family members to share details about the resident that will help staff understand the person in their care better. Inquire about possible concerns family members may have and learn what areas of care are of high importance to them. Discuss options that would make the resident happy, such as eating lunch outside on a warm summer day or having a bird feeder outside his or her window. These types of comforting choices enhance the living experience for residents and help them feel at home. Engaging and involving the family also strengthens the relationship with the caregiver and leads to positive outcomes for everyone involved.

Neighborhoods may have other visitors throughout the course of the day, such as supply delivery persons, physical therapists, dietitians, social workers, chaplains, hospice workers, physicians, and so forth. These personnel also contribute to the daily lives of residents and visit often. Sometimes, however, the flow of unfamiliar traffic makes residents uncomfortable. Dedicated staff should form relationships with these personnel to ensure the atmosphere remains home-like and comfortable and to put the residents at ease. Staff should be welcoming, cordial, and willing to assist outside personnel as they perform their jobs to benefit the residents. Staff should introduce the visitors to residents and explain their purpose or function. All visitors should be educated on the importance of maintaining a person-centered environment and encouraged to be respectful of the residents' home.

To foster communication with residents, staff can use conversation starters during care, at meal time, and throughout the course of the day. They can ask questions such as the following:

- What did you enjoy most about your favorite car?
- What were some fun things you did on your favorite vacation?
- What was interesting about your former career or favorite job?
- Who do you admire?
- What accomplishments are you most proud of?
- What is your favorite Bible verse?

Bring in magazines or books that encourage lively conversation, such as on travel or cooking. Involve the residents in turning pages and reading passages. Remember to allow ample time for the residents to react and respond to your questions. It may take them time to comprehend, remember, and phrase their responses. It is acceptable to help residents' complete thoughts or sentences if it appears they are searching for the right words. Keep a relaxed pace and do not hurry them along; this will only frustrate them, and inevitably they will give up. Reminiscing can bring comfort and joy to their day and help create relationships with caregivers.

Building relationships between team members and residents is person-centered care personified. The bonds that are created often continue for years and are the difference between truly enjoying your career and just working at a job for a paycheck. Your residents deserve the best care possible to enhance their lives, feel connected to the community, and maintain their personhood.

Building Successful Relationships
REVIEW

- Building relationships with residents helps staff provide person-centered care.

- Create a personalized environment to build a home-like atmosphere for residents.

- Interview residents to learn their personal preferences.

- Share tidbits of appropriate personal information to help enhance relationships with residents.

- Engage family members in the relationship-building process and invite their input.

- Welcome visitors and build relationships with them to help maintain the residents' peaceful, home-like environment.

- Use conversation starters to engage residents in reminiscing and to evoke happy memories.

- A trusting and caring environment leads to positive outcomes for residents.

NOTES

_____

_____

_____

_____

_____

_____

_____

The Story of Me

RESIDENT NAME _____

ROOM # _____ ADMISSION DATE _____

By what name do you prefer to be called? _____

What time do you like to rise in the morning? _____

What time do you like to go to bed? _____

Do you like to take naps during the day? _____

What time do you prefer to have your meals? _____

Do you have any religious dietary restrictions, such as not eating meat on Fridays or eating

kosher foods? _____

Are there special foods you like to eat at holidays? _____

How often do you prefer to bathe each week? _____

Do you prefer a shower, tub bath, or whirlpool bath? _____

Do you have any favorite items, such as a particular sweater or blanket? _____

_____

Do you prefer your room bright or dimly lit? _____

Are there any cultural or religious considerations you would like to have accommodated? _____

_____

Are there any hobbies or crafts you enjoy doing? _____

How do you prefer to spend your spare time? _____

Do you like a certain type of music? _____

Do you like sports? _____

Are there any games you like to play, such as card or board games? _____

_____

Is there anything you would like the staff to know to help them in providing care for you? _____

_____

Enhancing Staff Retention in Person-Centered Care Environments for Older Adults: How to Create and Implement a Comprehensive Orientation Program, by Janine M. Lange. Copyright © 2016 by Health Professions Press, Inc. All rights reserved. www.healthpropress.com.

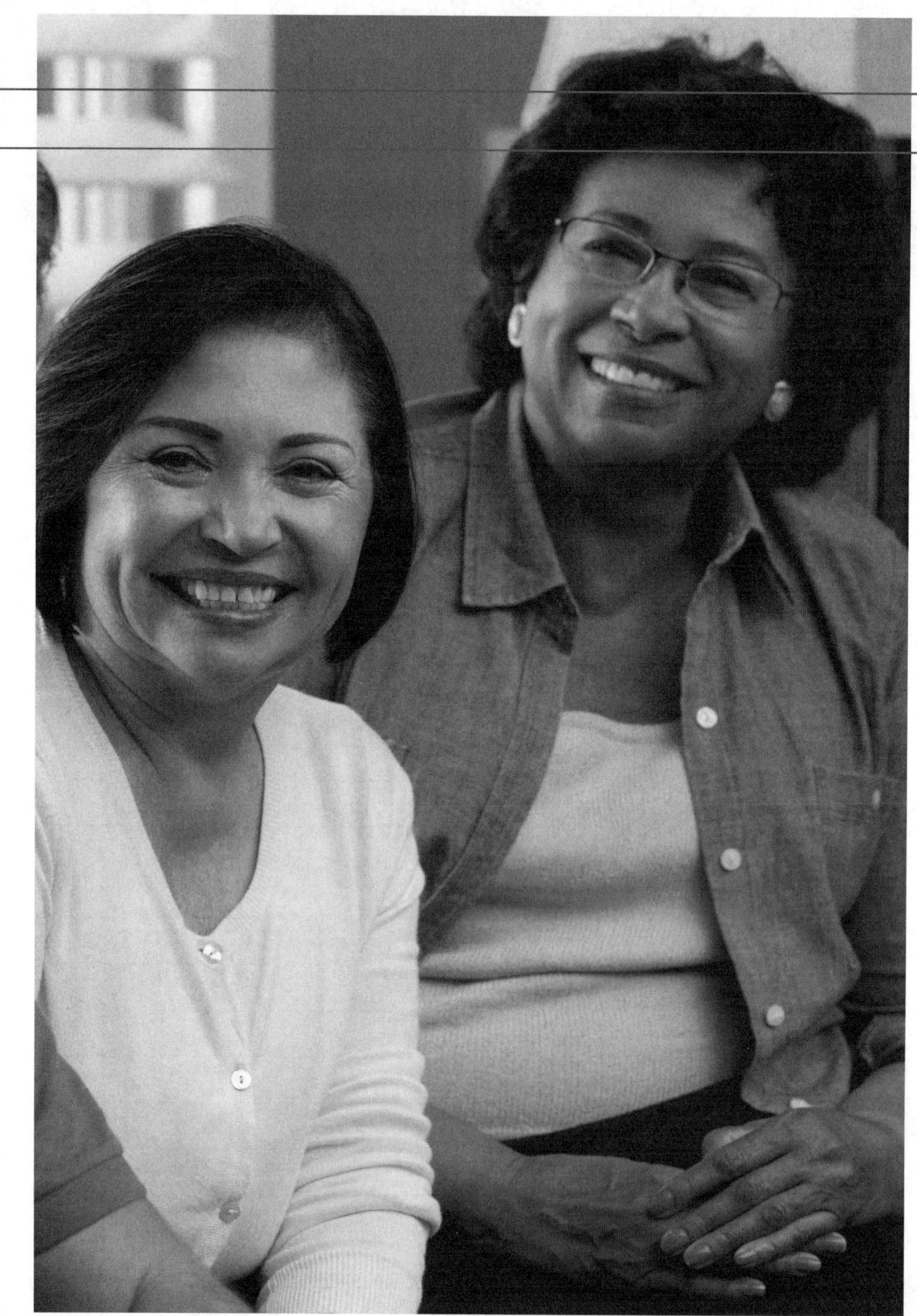

CHAPTER 9

Celebrating Diversity

It is important to recognize and welcome cultural diversity when new team members join your community. Their cultural traditions and customs will be diverse and unique, and some new staff will not be fluent in English. Potential barriers exist when an accent makes it difficult for someone to be understood, when idioms are not recognized, and when cultural differences lead to misunderstandings. Anticipating during the staff orientation process how to help keep potential issues from becoming challenges can reap benefits down the road. You must strive to show orientees for whom English is a second language that you are willing to assist them with any language barriers they may be experiencing to help them communicate effectively with residents, their families, and other staff members. Additionally, and in keeping with a person-centered care focus, your community should acknowledge the traditions and customs that residents and staff observe, to strengthen the relationship-building process between staff and residents and among team members.

Residents will appreciate your openness when introducing new team members who may speak English as a second language and with a heavy accent . For example, you may begin a conversation by saying, "Good morning, Mrs. Green. I am so happy to introduce you to the newest member of the nursing team. Her name is Rosella and she is from the Philippines. She comes to our community with a lot of experience and we are very excited to have her here." Allow the new nurse to engage in conversation with the resident and assess the resident's degree of comprehension. If the resident is having difficulty understanding the nurse, you may add, "Rosella speaks with a beautiful accent, and if you are having any trouble understanding her, I will be more than happy to translate for you until you two become better acquainted." This will help put both the resident and the new nurse at ease from the start and set the stage for mutual respect and understanding. Over time as a resident gets to know a new team member better, he or she will become accustomed to the person's speech patterns and both the resident and new hire will have no problems communicating.

There are several ways you can help address potential barriers to communication with any new team members for whom English is a second language. One solution is to have interpreters available who can assist in translating conversations between staff and residents. Poll your staff to determine if any team members speak a language other than English and enlist them to serve as interpreters. If your community has combined levels of care, such as independent and assisted living, you may ask residents from those Neighborhoods to serve as volunteers to help translate for residents who are experiencing difficulties communicating with a new team member. Encouraging interactions among residents from various levels of care enhances person-centered care.

Team members who speak the same language can help each other translate and share ways to communicate. This also helps build teamwork and fellowship among staff. Set aside some time for a team to meet, share their experiences, and discuss methods of communication they have found to be effective. Offer recommendations, such as speaking slowly and clearly until they have a better grasp of the English language and grammar, which will help them to be better understood by residents and other staff members.

Your community may be able to offer classes in basic English pronunciation and grammar, either in person or by podcast or webinar. There are also useful basic English lessens posted to YouTube.com that you may want to recommend to new team members who want to review and practice on their own. Most community colleges also offer ESL classes (English as a second language). Perhaps your organization can offer scholarships or tuition reimbursement for staff who attend these classes. There are also websites and phone and tablet apps available that translate any language into English.

During the orientation program, offer to spend a little extra time with new team members who may be experiencing difficulty in completing the necessary paperwork and forms. Explain the purpose of the forms and any implied expectations they may include, such as wearing a gait belt as part of their uniform. Be sure also to review the guidelines for absenteeism.

For documentation, use pictures or graphics to help staff understand how to chart correctly. Some electronic medical record (EMR) systems have illustrations of simple ADL (activities of daily living) functions built into their programs, such as for brushing teeth, showering, or bathing. If your EMR does not include graphics, create a "cheat sheet" and display it near the computer where the team performs their charting. Give staff their own copy on which they can write personal notes.

Examples of basic illustrations to assist in charting can be found at the end of the chapter.

It is equally important to encourage your staff to be cognizant of the religious or cultural traditions of residents. An example would be a resident who uses rosary beads for daily prayer. New team members need to be instructed that the rosary beads should be readily available and within reach. Review each resident's care plan and *The Story of Me* with new staff to ensure they honor and respect each person's preferences. Likewise, extend to staff members the opportunity to share their cultural customs and traditions. Plan a special luncheon or brunch to celebrate holidays that are significant to staff from other countries. Invite team members to prepare traditional foods and to decorate according to their customs. Encourage staff to dress in cultural attire, if they choose to. The occasion can be used as a group activity by involving residents, and can help build relationships on the Neighborhood. Celebrations and holidays are the moments that enrich our lives, deepen our sense of heritage, and create happy memories. By sharing cultural and religious traditions, the care team and residents learn how to understand and relate to each other. Person-centered care is embodied in the interactions between caregivers and residents and their families and is strengthened when joyous moments are shared together.

A culturally diverse care team brings together an assorted blend of individuals. No matter what language your team members speak, they all share the same intentions and common goals of providing person-centered care to residents. By acknowledging the cultural or language differences of staff and residents and helping them to overcome communication obstacles, you create a caring Neighborhood built on respect and mutual admiration.

Celebrating Diversity
REVIEW

- Identify language barriers new team members may have.
- Introduce new staff with accents or dialects to residents and help them get acquainted with each other.
- Seek out translators or interpreters within the community and enlist their help.
- Build teamwork by encouraging staff with similar backgrounds to help each other.
- Offer ESL classes or reimbursement for off-campus English education.
- Spend extra time reviewing paperwork during orientation with staff who are challenged in reading English.
- Use graphics or pictures to help new staff understand EMR documentation.
- Review the religious and cultural traditions of residents during care plan meetings.
- Celebrate the cultural traditions of staff and include residents.

NOTES

_____

_____

_____

_____

_____

_____

_____

Sample EMR Graphics to Assist with Charting

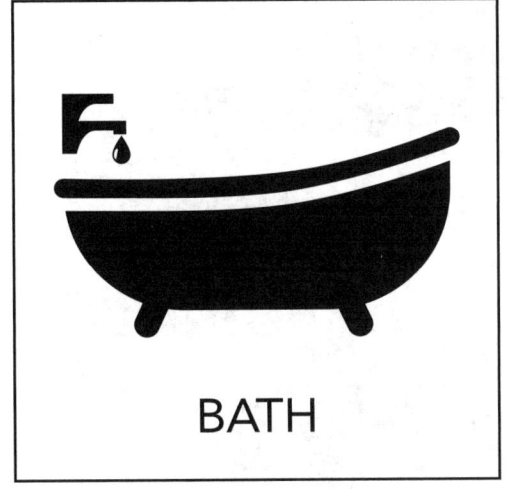

BATH

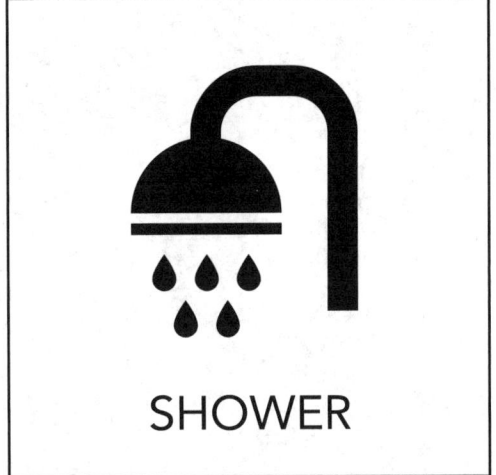

SHOWER

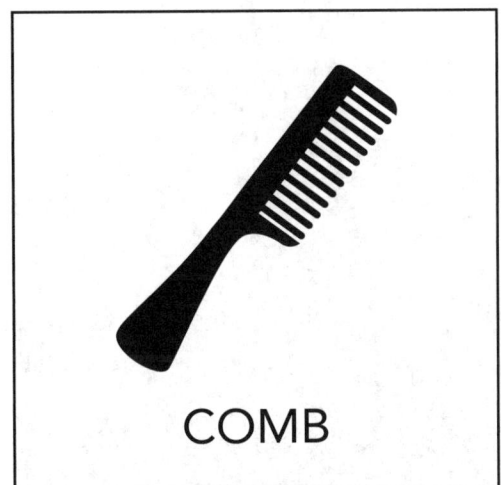

COMB

BRUSH

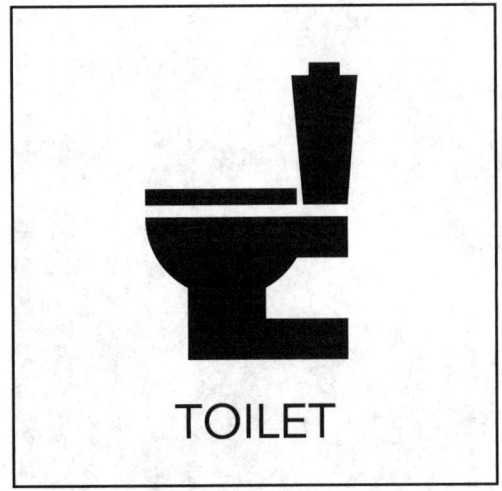

TOILET

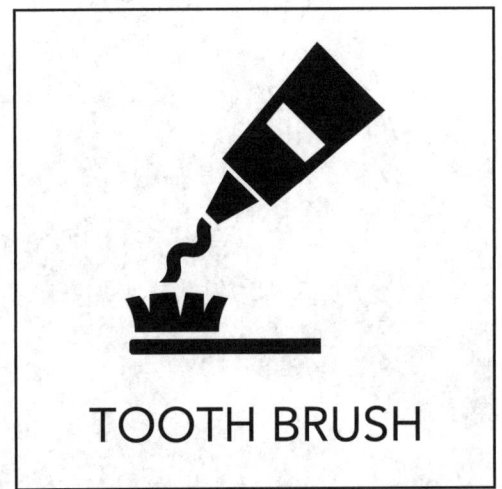

TOOTH BRUSH

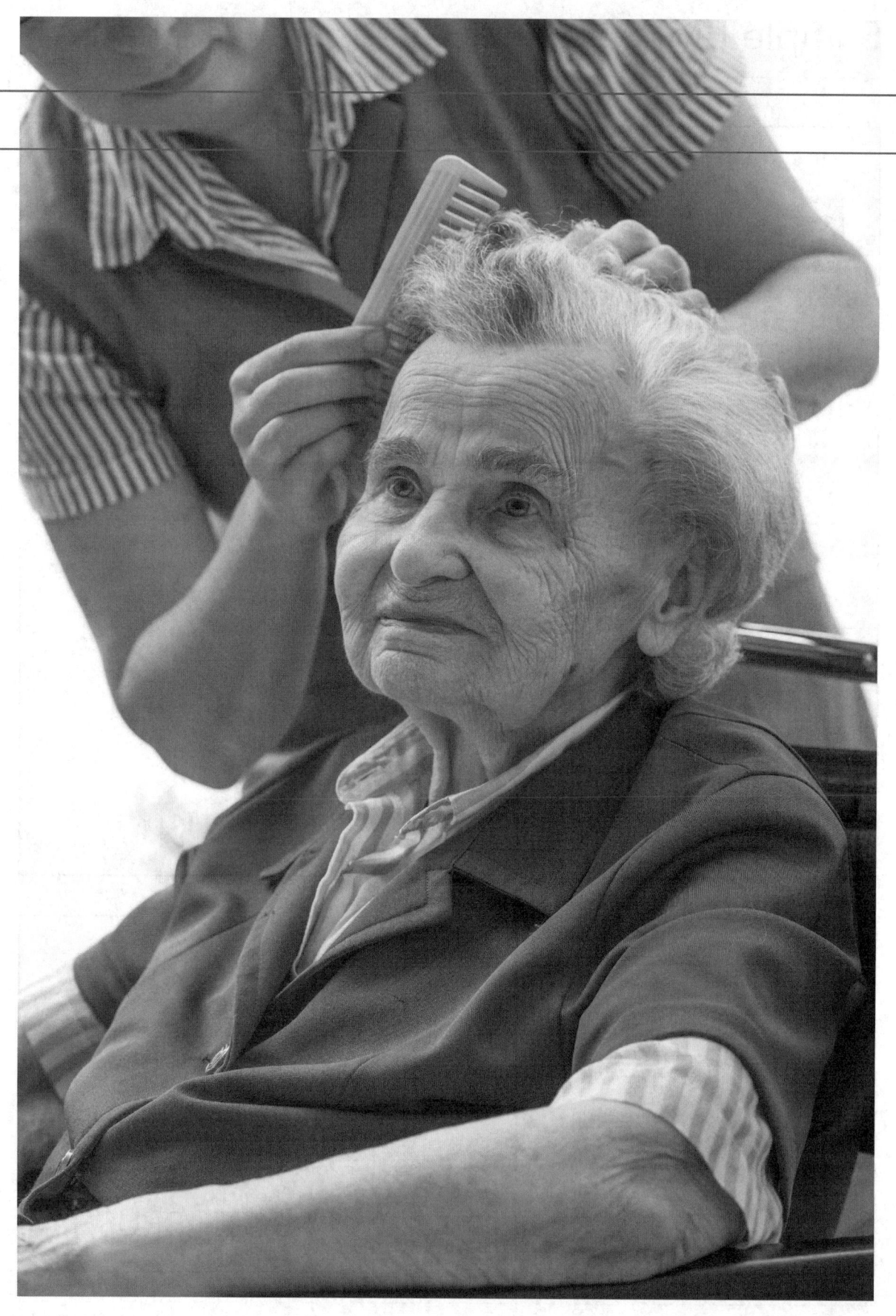

CHAPTER 10

Showing You Care

The first few days and weeks on the Neighborhood will prove to be the most challenging for new team members. It is important to reassure them that many people are looking out for them. New team members work alongside their mentors daily until the orientation period has ended, but what about contact with other team members? The nursing supervisor, director of nursing (DON), nurse educator, and fellow co-workers should interact with new hires on a daily basis to offer support and encouragement. The direct supervisor should be in touch with an orientee every day for at least the first week and every other day for the second week and should ask questions such as the following:

- How are things going?
- Are you comfortable with your mentor?
- Do you feel you are learning what you need to in order to perform your duties?
- Do you have any questions or concerns I can address?
- Is there anything you need?

Maintaining a connection and line of communication with the new team members makes them feel welcomed and cared about. If they are having any conflicts with their mentors or feel they are unable to learn from them, the supervisor needs to know this information early on to prevent unfavorable outcomes. If the orientees feel uncomfortable bringing this information to the supervisor's attention, asking them directly how things are going with their mentor may help them to convey their concerns without feeling intimidated.

If an orientee and mentor are not working well together, it is important to assign a new mentor immediately. Let the orientee know it is certainly not a problem to change mentors and that you appreciate his or her being honest and forthright. The mentors should expect to encounter times when conflicting personalities or learning styles prevent a positive mentoring experience. Both parties should act professionally and continue to be amicable toward each other.

The nurse educator, or whoever conducted the orientation program, should also be making contact with a new team member on a regular basis. For the first 2 to 3 weeks, he or she should make sure an orientee is becoming acclimated to the Neighborhood as well as be available as a resource to answer any questions the new hire may have. Also, the educator should make sure all of the passwords and user IDs issued during the orientation are working and that an orientee has full access to the electronic charting and any websites he or she may need to visit, such as the pharmacy or lab. The educator can also offer to provide a 60- to 90-minute refresher class on any topics the orientee feels he or she requires more education on. Information overload is sure to occur during the first few days of orientation, so offering some individual training can help a new team member if he or she is feeling overwhelmed.

The DON should also be making contact with a new team member at least once or twice during the first few weeks. This truly sends the message that each member of the team is important and that his or her contribution to the Neighborhood is valued. This is a great time to spend a few minutes together to get to know each other and begin to form a relationship in keeping with the person-centered focus of the community. It also helps the DON stay connected to the staff and build mutual trust. If and when a new team member has a concern or suggestion, he or she should feel comfortable approaching the DON as opposed to only interacting with him or her when something negative has occurred. An open-door policy keeps the lines of communication open and helps the DON gain insight into potential problems that may be preventing the team from delivering excellent care to residents.

Encourage other members of the team, especially from different departments, such as homemakers, housekeepers, dining aides, and so forth, to interact with new team members. A housekeeper or laundry assistant can show them where to discard soiled linens and where to get clean linens. Dining aides can help show them which residents like to sit at which tables, who their tablemates usually are, and the mealtime preferences of individual residents. This is a person-centered approach to building the team; everyone is involved in the orientation process to make the new team members feel welcomed and at home in the Neighborhood.

After the first 2 to 3 weeks as a new team member begins to feel comfortable and at ease in the Neighborhood, the supervisor may only need to touch base with him or her once a week. This will keep the lines of communication open and give the supervisor a chance to observe the orientee's interaction with the residents and other team members.

It is a good practice for the nurse educator to reassemble the orientation group after the first 30 days for a review and evaluation of their progress. At this point, the new team members have been actively working for 4 weeks and have a better understanding of their roles. If there are any procedures that are unclear or areas of concern that need to be addressed, the review will give them the perfect arena to ask questions without feeling embarrassed or intimidated. Meeting again also strengthens the relationship with the educator and helps team members feel comfortable in utilizing him or her as a resource. Of course, the new team member should feel free to visit the educator or instructor at any time, but a formal invitation to discuss any issues he or she may be experiencing is always welcomed and appreciated.

The length of time a new team member will require for orientation is determined on an individual basis. There are several factors to be considered when deciding if the new team member is ready to work independently, including the following:

- amount and type of prior experience

- ability to demonstrate skills accurately and appropriately

- understanding of and integration into the culture of the community

- ability to work well with co-workers

- degree of initiative and desire to work independently

Those who should be involved in the decision-making process are the mentor, orientee, and direct supervisor. The mentor will provide the most input in determining the orientee's readiness to work independently by using the skills demonstration checklists and his or her observations as guides. If the mentor feels strongly that the orientee is not yet able to safely and independently perform the duties, he or she should express that to the supervisor at this time and recommend extending the mentoring period.

It is important for the new team member to feel comfortable in transitioning from working under the guidance of a mentor to fully taking on his or her new role. Although the mentor will still be available to provide guidance and support when needed, the expectation once the mentoring period has ended is that the new team member is able to work independently. If he or she expresses reservations, ask the orientee why he or she feels that way and what type of additional support or instruction he or she requires. Set a mutually agreeable amount of time for more training or mentoring. Meet again at the end of the extended orientation period to determine if the time allotted was sufficient.

The supervisor should meet with the new team member and the mentor individually to hear each person's thoughts and opinions on whether the orientation period should be extended. The supervisor's first priority is to ensure the safety and security of the residents and the cohesion of the care team. Ultimately, the supervisor should make the final decision based on the input received from the mentor and orientee.

Showing you care and are genuinely concerned about the success of new team members will have lasting effects and far-reaching benefits. For the orientee, he or she will feel at ease, accepted, and more apt to have an open and honest relationship with the residents as well as his or her co-workers and supervisors. This will, in turn, help nursing leadership build a reliable and dedicated team. The residents will reap the benefits of being provided loving care from a consistent and dependable team of caregivers. Ultimately, the care you show for your staff will spread throughout your community.

Showing You Care

REVIEW

- The mentor and other team members should have daily contact with new team members during their first 2 weeks on the Neighborhood.

- Direct supervisors, DONs, and nurse educators should be in close contact with orientees often during the first few weeks.

- The mentor should ask the new team member questions to determine how well things are going and to assess if changes are needed to the orientation process.

- Each department can be a part of the orientation process.

- The nurse educator should reassemble with new team members after the first 4 weeks on the Neighborhood to review and evaluate their progress.

- The mentor, orientee, and nursing supervisor determine the length of time of the orientation period and whether to extend it.

NOTES

_____

_____

_____

_____

_____

_____

_____

_____

_____

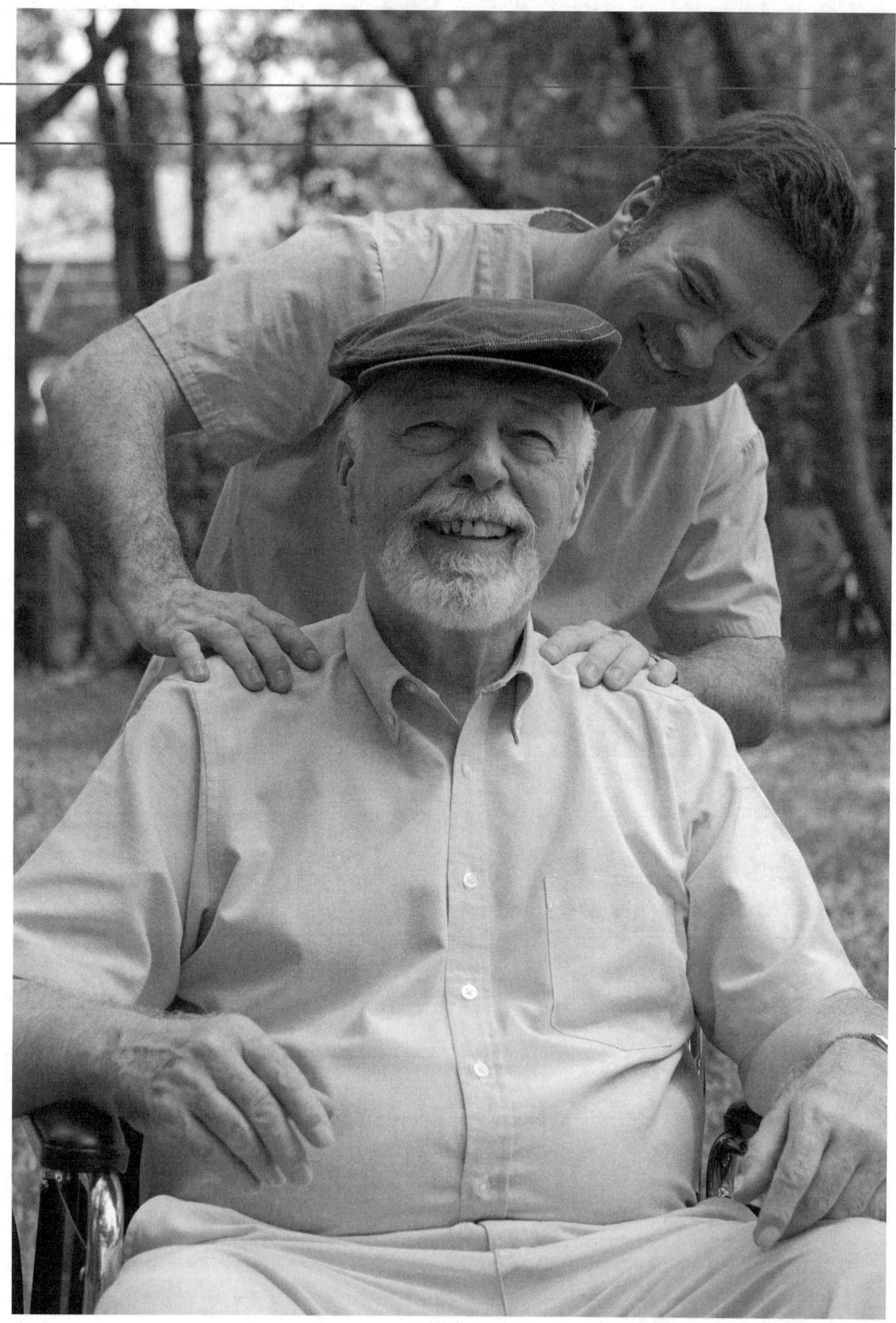

CHAPTER 11

Evaluations

Evaluations are essential tools to help gauge the effectiveness of the orientation program and assess the need for changes and improvements. Soliciting feedback from new team members who have actually taken part in the program from beginning to end can give you an insider's point of view as to which portions of the program are successful and which need to be improved. The information gathered from the evaluations should be shared with everyone involved in presenting information as part of the orientation program. The nursing leadership team should meet to discuss whether the goals of the program are being met as well as brainstorm new and better methods of education.

When building your evaluations, keep in mind the main objectives of the orientation program and devise questions to help determine if they have been met. Evaluations are performed at different times throughout the orientation process. There are two evaluations that should be a part of the orientation program:

- *Nursing Orientation Evaluation:* Conducted immediately after the general nursing orientation has been completed
- *30-to-60-Day Mentorship Evaluation:* Completed 30 to 60 days after the new hire has had time to work in the Neighborhood alongside a mentor

The Nursing Orientation Evaluation should be conducted following the initial 1- or 2-day general nursing orientation to assess that portion of the training. The evaluation form should be distributed and completed directly following the end of class so the information is fresh in each orientee's mind. The evaluation asks basic questions relative to the program content and the instructor. Although the orientees are not yet able to answer questions related to their specific duties, you will want to know how well the initial segment was received by them. The questions should pertain to the manner in which the program was presented, the use of audio/visual aids, the effectiveness and knowledge of the speaker or speakers, and whether the orientees have an understanding of their role in a person-centered care environment. The evaluation form is completed anonymously and turned in to the immediate supervisor of the person conducting the class. A numerical value is given to each answer since the questions do not require in-depth answers. The bottom of the evaluation form includes a section for additional comments and suggestions. The nurse supervisor will share the information with other members of the nursing leadership team as well as with the program presenters and make recommendations based on the findings. At the end of the chapter is a sample Nursing Orientation Evaluation Form for a 2-day class.

The 30-to-60-Day Mentorship Evaluation should be completed after the orientee has had time to learn his or her new job working alongside a mentor in the Neighborhood (30 to 60 days after the mentoring period had been completed). Depending on how many shifts the orientee has actually worked, you can decide, in consultation with the mentor and orientee, when within the 30 to 60 days the evaluation can be completed. The questions address the usefulness of information provided during the orientation process, how well the mentor experience is progressing, and if the orientee feels he or she is integrating well into the culture of the community. The evaluation form is not graded numerically because open-ended questions are asked that require written feedback. Depending on the policies of your organization regarding a probationary period, this evaluation can serve as a good assessment of whether an orientee is qualified to assume a permanent status by the end of the probation period. Based on the findings of the evaluation, the mentor has time to work with the orientee to address any areas that need improvement and to observe whether additional education efforts were successful. Input from the mentor and other staff who have interacted with the new team member will be beneficial in making the determination to hire the orientee permanently after the 90-day probationary period. A sample 30-to-60-Day Mentorship Evaluation Form can be found at the end the chapter.

The nursing leadership team should meet periodically to discuss whether the goals set for new team members are being met, and the rate of employee retention should be tracked. If your community is part of a larger organization, it is good practice to network with leaders of sister communities to share ideas and create a standardized method of education throughout the organization.

The ultimate goal of any healthcare organization is to provide residents safe, efficient, and high-quality care. Maintaining resident choice is paramount to delivering person-centered care. Building a dedicated, well-trained staff is one of the key steps for achieving these goals. Residents will thrive, families will be satisfied with the care and attention their loved one is receiving, and new and existing staff will excel as they attain greater confidence in their capabilities.

The evaluations that are a part of the orientation period are essential to ensuring new hires are adapting well to working on the Neighborhood, including learning and following the community's processes and procedures. The annual state survey will provide the definitive proof that the processes and procedures in place are sound and effective, and a deficiency-free survey will show that all standards of care as mandated by the state are being met. The nursing leadership team, however, is responsible for creating a system that will meet or exceed mandated standards as well as the community's planned goals by incorporating person-centered care practices, capable staff, fiduciary responsibility, and, above all, a caring and loving environment for those whom they serve. There are, however, potential barriers in successfully training new team members and incorporating them into the community, which Chapter 12 discusses.

Evaluations
REVIEW

- Evaluations are an essential component in gauging the effectiveness of an orientation program.

- Evaluation questions correlate to the stage of new-hire training completed.

- Information from the evaluations is quantified by the instructor conducting the orientation program and reviewed by the nursing leadership team.

- The instructor shares the evaluation results with his or her immediate supervisor, the nursing leadership team, program presenters, and leaders in sister communities.

- The nursing leadership team recommends changes, revisions, and additions to the program based on evaluation feedback.

- Employee retention rates and annual state surveys are key indicators of successful outcomes in building a dedicated, well-trained staff.

NOTES

_____

_____

_____

_____

_____

_____

_____

_____

_____

Nursing Orientation Evaluation Form

CLASS *Nursing Clinical Orientation*

NAME OF TRAINER _____

DATE _____

Your feedback is very important. Please provide your thoughts and comments about the orientation program so we can continue to develop training that best suits your needs as well as those of future new team members. Thank you in advance for your opinions!

Using the following guide, please circle the appropriate number for each of the questions below:

Not at all		Somewhat		Completely
1	2	3	4	5

1. I have a good understanding of what is expected of me in my new role.

   1   2   3   4   5

2. I have a good understanding of culture change and person-centered care.

   1   2   3   4   5

3. Content was presented in an organized manner.

   1   2   3   4   5

4. Content was presented clearly and effectively.

   1   2   3   4   5

5. The presenter was responsive to questions/comments.

   1   2   3   4   5

6. Teaching aids/audiovisuals were used effectively.

   1   2   3   4   5

7. Teaching style was effective.

   1   2   3   4   5

8. Content met stated objectives.

   1   2   3   4   5

9. Content presented was applicable to my practice.

   1   2   3   4   5

30- to 60-Day Mentorship Evaluation Form

NAME _____

TITLE _____

DATE OF HIRE _____

DATE COMPLETED _____

It has been 30 to 60 days since your orientation class. We would like your feedback on your experience working in your Neighborhood/Household since that time. Please answer the following questions as completely and honestly as possible so we may better serve your needs and those of future new team members.

1. Was the information presented during the Nursing Department Orientation appropriate and useful?

   _____

   _____

2. Do you feel you were provided enough information to perform your job well? If not, what do you feel should have been included?

   _____

   _____

3. What information presented during the Nursing Department Orientation was most beneficial to you in your new role?

   _____

   _____

4. What information presented during the Nursing Department Orientation was least beneficial to you in your new role?

   _____

   _____

continued

30- to 60-Day Mentorship Evaluation Form *cont.*

NAME _____

5. Was there anything that you feel you needed to know that was not presented?

    _____

    _____

6. How do you feel you fit in with the culture of the community?

    _____

    _____

7. Do you feel you received adequate training and support from your Mentor?

    _____

    _____

8. Do you feel you received adequate training and support from your Clinical Nurse Leader?

    _____

    _____

9. Please provide comments on how you feel your orientation experience could have been better.

    _____

    _____

10. Please provide your comments on how the orientation process benefited your transition into your new position.

    _____

    _____

Thank you for your time and participation!

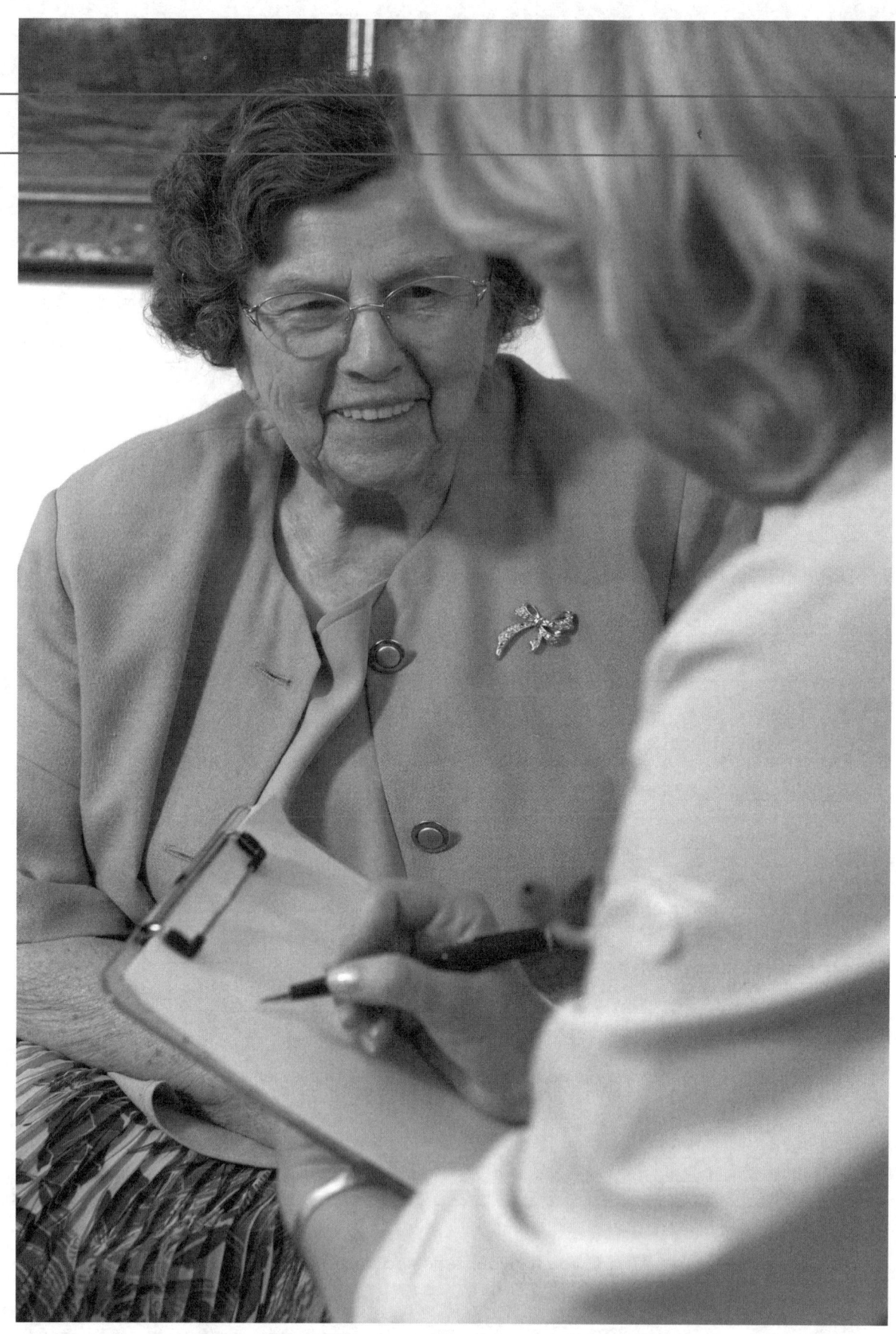

CHAPTER 12

Barriers to Success

As new team members come aboard, it is important to set the stage for success and build a long-lasting relationship with them. There are, however, obstacles that can prevent a new hire from starting off on the right foot and becoming a valuable part of the team. Being cognizant of the following five common barriers to success will help ensure that new hires can develop good relationships with residents and staff:

- Poor mentoring
- Inadequate training
- Lack of clearly defined expectations
- Skills not tested or enhanced
- Lack of follow up with new team members

POOR MENTORING

Mentoring is an area most often overlooked in training new hires. When communities are challenged with staffing, it is tempting to place a new team member with the first available person who may or may not be a good fit. The mentor role should be thoughtfully considered and planned well in advance of a new hire's first day. As discussed in Chapter 3, when choosing mentors, begin with an application and interview process. Require staff to apply for a mentoring position with the recommendation of their supervisor. During the interview process, pay close attention to the applicant's work ethic, punctuality, interpersonal skills, and ability to teach. Not every good employee is a good teacher; therefore, make sure the applicant is comfortable in the role of mentor. Mentors should be very enthusiastic about their job, their employer, and the opportunity to welcome new staff to the team. The first impression made by a mentor will be a lasting one and will set the tone for the orientation experience.

Ideally, a pre-assigned mentor or partner should be the new team member's first point of contact when orientation into the Neighborhood begins. A time should be set up prior to the first actual work day for the two to meet and get acquainted. They should discuss when and where they will meet at the start of the shift. The mentor should relay important information that will help ease first-day anxieties, such as where to park, where to clock in, location of lockers, and so forth. Being greeted by a familiar face on the first day will lessen a new team member's anxiety and put him or her at ease in the new environment.

INADEQUATE TRAINING

Providing sufficient training prior to allowing a team member to work independently lays the groundwork for success. Some communities may feel there is not enough time for a dedicated training process or that any training should be done while on the job. Seriously consider how placing a poorly trained nurse or aide on an assignment can have significant negative outcomes for your residents, community, and staff.

Depending on a new team member's level of experience and background, the individual orientation timeframe will vary. A newly graduated nurse will need more time to acclimate to his or her new role in providing very basic levels of care, whereas a seasoned nurse with years of experience under his or her belt may require a more rudimentary orientation. Specific fields of nursing can also determine how much training is needed, such as an acute care nurse transitioning into a long-term care model. There are significant differences between the two environments, and ample time should be allowed to become accustomed to the changes. The supervisor, mentor, and new team member should mutually agree to the amount of time spent in orientation and training. A few extra days with a mentor, for example, can make a world of difference.

LACK OF CLEARLY DEFINED EXPECTATIONS

There should be no vagueness as to what actually is expected of a new team member. The direct supervisor, orientee, and mentor should meet together to discuss expectations once the nursing orientation program has been completed. It is always best to have a written agenda or outline clearly defining the job description (typically given to the new hire by the Human Resources department at the time of hire). Discuss each point together and answer any questions that arise completely, succinctly, and without ambiguity. By painting a clear picture of the duties that are to be performed, the orientee cannot say, "I didn't know I was supposed to do that." Have the orientee sign the detailed list and provide him or her with a copy. Be sure to lend your support and encourage the new team member to take advantage of the orientation time period to learn as much as possible about his or her new role in the community.

Skills Not Tested or Enhanced

As discussed in Chapter 6, skills testing should be done across the board regardless of a staff member's experience or background. It is the only concrete way to assess proficiency and accuracy in demonstrating various skills related to a specific discipline. For experienced personnel, it is a way to review and enhance skills as well as correct poor habits that have been learned over time. For new team members, skills testing is a way to assess their readiness to begin working independently on the Neighborhood. In addition to skills testing, a community should offer ongoing skills training for all staff.

Create a skills checklist for each discipline that addresses each scope of practice accordingly. Depending on your community's policies and procedures, you can also customize a skills checklist to suit your needs. In skills testing new hires, demonstrate proper techniques and have each orientee perform a return demonstration as part of the orientation period.

Medication administration is an area of skills testing that should be given considerable attention with new team members. If your community uses certified medication technicians (CMTs) for medication passes, you must clearly define their scope of practice within your community's guidelines. For example, state whether CMTs are allowed to perform glucose testing and administer insulin, even if they are certified to do so. Some communities prefer to have only licensed nurses administer and monitor insulin.

Depending on the types of medications typically used and the scope of practice for the nurses and CMTs, each community is required to test CMTs as well as LPNs and RNs on medication administration in the form of a written exam and a return demonstration. The written test should contain questions that are specific to both the general and geriatric populations and within each discipline's scope of practice. To ensure your test has the most current methods of medication administration, enlist your long-term care pharmacy as a resource to provide up-to-date policies and procedures. The Centers for Disease Control and Prevention is another good source of current information.

Create a set of orders that includes all types of medications (e.g., oral, ophthalmological, IV, rectal, patches, nebulizers, etc.), and test new staff on the proper procedure for administration, monitoring, and documentation as well as for addressing potential adverse reactions. Encourage staff to openly discuss past experiences, both positive and negative, that can impact administering medication accurately.

LACK OF FOLLOW UP WITH NEW TEAM MEMBERS

Following up with new team members is important for many reasons. It is essential to make sure they are comfortable in and adjusting to their new environment as well as adapting to the culture of the Neighborhood. Additionally, by remaining in close contact with new team members in the first few days and weeks of employment you are demonstrating the following:

- Person-centered care encompasses not only the residents, but the staff as well.

- You are investing time and resources in new staff because it is important that you give them the tools needed to be successful in their new roles.

- Each individual is essential to the success of the team and will be provided the necessary resources to perform his or her job well.

Barriers to Success

REVIEW

- Set new team members up for success by developing and supporting a mentoring component to the orientation process.

- Create an enthusiastic and welcoming environment for new hires.

- Allow the orientee and mentor to mutually decide on the training period.

- Clearly define expectations from the start.

- Test skills at the beginning of employment.

- Regularly make contact with new team members.

NOTES

_____

_____

_____

_____

_____

_____

_____

_____

_____

_____

_____

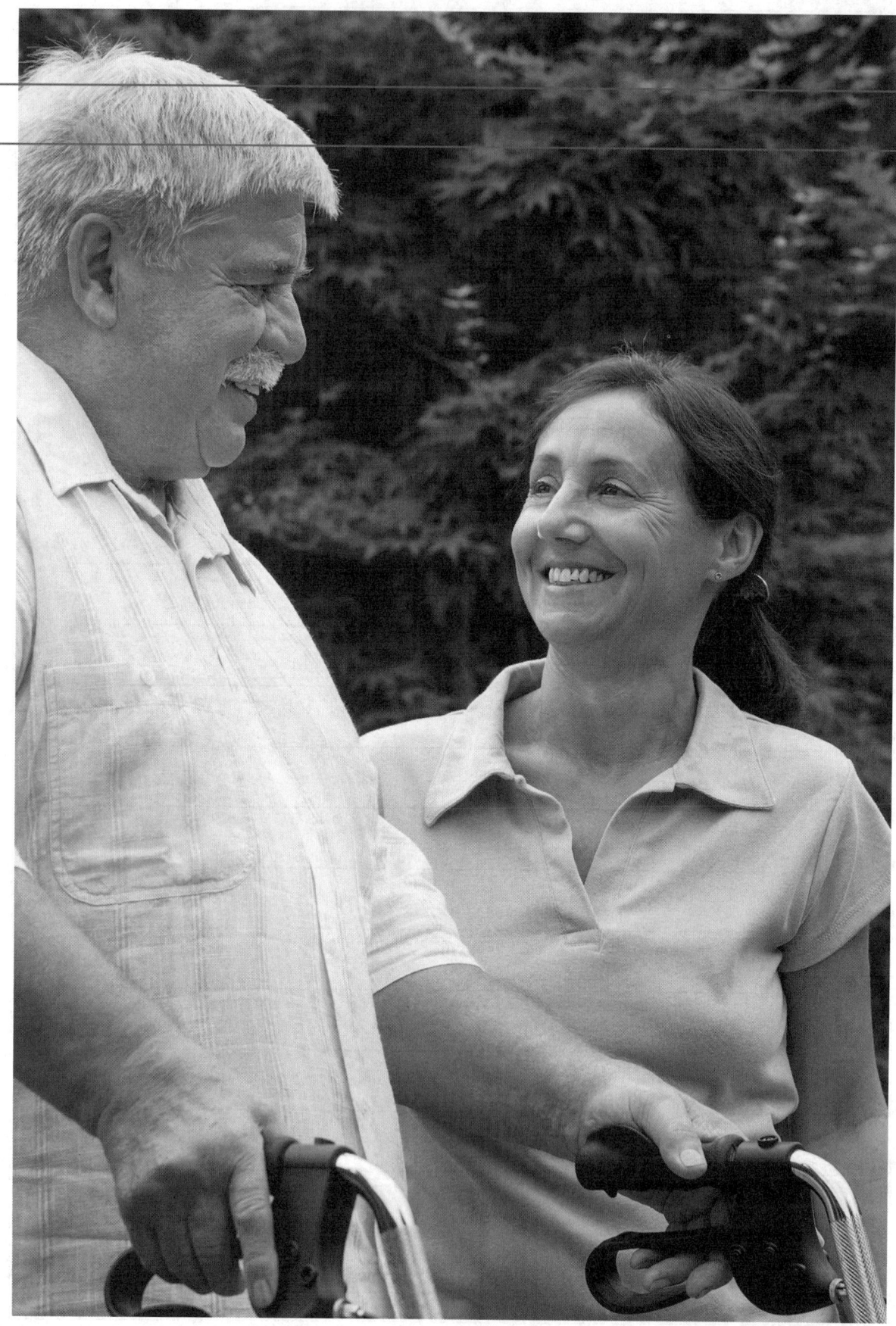

CHAPTER 13

Person-Centered Care
The Heart of the Matter

Establishing a comprehensive orientation program is one of the best ways to promote and maintain a person-centered community. The benefits of a well-trained team of dedicated staff are far reaching and long lasting. Confident team members take pride in their work and devote their time to providing excellent care to residents. The residents feel safe, secure, and loved in their homes. Families can feel assured that their loved ones are being cared for just as they would do so. Others who have the opportunity to visit or conduct business in the community, such as physicians, adjunct care providers, and vendors, will immediately notice a well-run, loving environment.

For new team members joining the community, it is encouraging to be embraced in a person-centered atmosphere. Witnessing how staff treat residents and each other in a positive, respectful manner is inspiring and motivates them to strive toward being good employees. The orientation program helps them transition into their new roles with ease and makes them feel welcomed by giving them time to learn as much as possible with the help of mentors, team leaders, and co-workers.

Share the following vignette with your new team members as a way to motivate and help them understand that residents' needs are at the heart of all they do:

Today is the first day of your new relationship with everyone in this community. Everything is new. The sights, sounds, and smells all seem a little foreign to you. When you walk throughout the community, it's easy to get lost because everywhere you go seems unfamiliar to you. When you sit down to eat lunch, all of the people at the table are strangers. When the phone rings, you are unsure of how to answer it because you don't remember the name of your Neighborhood. If someone asks for the phone or fax number, you haven't yet learned either and cannot answer. You have been introduced to so many people and cannot possibly remember all of their names or what they do each day. You feel a little embarrassed because your mentor has tried to explain a new concept to you two or three times but it just doesn't make any sense to you yet. You move more slowly through processes than the other team members because you are still learning new procedures. There are so many things to remember that is seems to be too much, and you have an overwhelming feeling to run away and escape. When it is time to leave, you cannot remember where the parking lot is or how to get there. At the end of the day you are exhausted, confused, and frustrated, and you fear that your job will never make sense to you.

In about 3 or 4 weeks, things are beginning to come together. You have started establishing a routine. You know exactly where to go and how to get there. People around you are becoming familiar and you call them by their name. It takes less time to think of how to perform your duties than it did just a few weeks ago. You are beginning to feel confident about working independently. At the end of the day, you feel satisfied and content that you did a good job and helped make someone's day a little brighter.

For the residents in your care, however, every day is the first day. They have difficulty remembering who you are, even though you were with them just yesterday. The faces of their tablemates for lunch are unfamiliar to them, regardless of the fact that they have eaten all of their meals together for months or years. They cannot remember what time or day it is, even if they were just told or if there is a clock or calendar on the wall. They get lost just walking back to their room and sometimes wander to places they shouldn't go. They walk slower, talk slower, and ask you to repeat things many times before finally giving up on trying to understand you. At the end of the day they feel tired, confused, lonely, depressed, frustrated, and afraid. The difference is, they will never catch on. Each day will bring despair and it will not improve as time goes on; in fact, it will most likely worsen with each day. But they have you to help them, care for them, encourage and support them, and make their lives better.

Remembering what it felt like those first few days and weeks of your job when you were new will help you relate to the residents' feelings and be understanding and compassionate. You can put yourself in their shoes and treat them the same way you were treated when you were new. You will be patient and loving when it appears a resident cannot do the simplest of tasks and will not rush him or her through the process. Instead, you will hold the resident's hand and let him or her know it is okay to take it slowly and move at his or her own pace. When residents are frightened you will comfort them, and when they are lonely you will provide companionship. When they are tired you will help attend to their needs. You will do this because you remember what your first day felt like and understand that for the resident every day is the first day.

And that is what person-centered care is all about—care for residents, staff, and all of those who we encounter each and every day.

Staff motivation can be derived from personal stories, life experiences, or examples of outstanding care provided by your team. Use cards and letters from satisfied residents and family members as a testimony to the excellent care the community is providing. The main goal is to create a person-centered care team who are dedicated to the residents and committed to making every minute of their lives the best they can be.

The orientation program will ensure your residents and staff are at the heart of your community's person-centered care approach. But even with a good orientation program and solid mentoring program, nothing takes the place of genuine compassion, kindness, and benevolence. As leaders, our priority is to set an example. We must show how to provide the best care possible by treating our residents, their loves ones, our colleagues, and our team members with dignity and respect as well as honor each individual's personhood. Putting out the welcome mat for new team members opens the door to a loving Neighborhood and helps continue the mission of providing person-centered care.

Person-Centered Care
REVIEW

- A good orientation program promotes and strengthens person-centered care.
- Team motivation and encouragement is essential to a successful orientation program.
- Inspire your new team members with personal stories.
- Cards and letters from satisfied residents and families validate your mission.
- Resident safety and satisfaction is the ultimate goal for a community in building a person-centered care team.
- Honor your residents and team of caregivers as part of your community's culture of person-centered care.

NOTES

_____

_____

_____

_____

_____

_____

_____

_____

_____

Index